# Clinical Pharmacology of Psychotherapeutic Drugs

## Third Edition

# Clinical Pharmacology of Psychotherapeutic Drugs

## Third Edition

### Leo E. Hollister, M.D.

Professor
Departments of Psychiatry and Behavioral Sciences and
 Pharmacology
University of Texas Medical School at Houston
Medical Director
Harris County Psychiatric Center
Houston, Texas

### John G. Csernansky, M.D.

Assistant Professor
Department of Psychiatry and Behavioral Sciences
Stanford University School of Medicine
Stanford, California

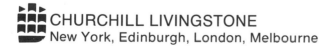 CHURCHILL LIVINGSTONE
New York, Edinburgh, London, Melbourne

**Library of Congress Cataloging-in-Publication Data**

Hollister, Leo E., date
    Clinical pharmacology of psychotherapeutic drugs. — 3rd ed. / Leo E.
Hollister, John G. Csernansky.
        p.    cm
    Includes bibliographical references.
    ISBN 0-443-08670-2
    1. Psychopharmacology.    2. Psychotropic drugs.    I. Csernansky,
John G.    II. Title
    [DNLM: 1. Hypnotics and Sedatives—pharmacology.    2. Psychotropic
Drugs—pharmacology.    QV 77 H744ca]
    RM315.H632    1990
    615'.78—dc20
    DNLM/DLC
    for Library of Congress                                    89-23847
                                                                 CIP

© **Churchill Livingstone Inc. 1990, 1983, 1978**

Distributed in the United Kingdom by Churchill Livingstone, Robert
Stevenson House, 1–3 Baxter's Place, Leith Walk, Edinburgh EH1 3AF,
and by associated companies, branches, and representatives throughout
the world.

Accurate indications, adverse reactions, and dosage schedules for drugs
are provided in this book, but it is possible that they may change. The
reader is urged to review the package information data of the
manufacturers of the medications mentioned.

The Publishers have made every effort to trace the copyright holders for
borrowed material. If they have inadvertently overlooked any, they will
be pleased to make the necessary arrangements at the first opportunity.

Acquisitions Editor: *Robert A. Hurley*
Copy Editor: *Elizabeth Bowman*
Production Designer: *Charlie Lebeda*

Printed in the United States of America

First published in 1990

# Preface to the Third Edition

Not long ago, I was looking up material in the textbook of psychiatry used when I was a student (actually I was trying to trace the concepts that have led to the currently popular diagnosis of panic disorder). The first edition of the book was published in the 1920s; the third edition, which our class used, was published in the early 1940s. Incredibly, not a word was changed in the section on anxiety disorders during that twenty-year period. Did it mean that no progress had been made in understanding or treating anxiety disorders during that period?

New editions of psychiatry books published today must be extensively rewritten, even when the span of time between editions is only a few years. Progress in understanding emotional disorders is rapid; progress in treating them is less rapid but by no means stationary. Concepts regarding both the cause and treatment of mental disorders change rapidly. Thus, this third edition of our book contains extensive re-writing from previous editions.

This edition has a new chapter describing the current use of drugs in children and adolescents. This area remains controversial, one might even say politicized, and definite rules are still uncertain. Nonetheless, it appears that many of these disorders may be amenable to drug treatment, even when it may not be the primary method of management.

Referencing articles or book chapters is highly idiosyncratic. Our approach has been to cite more recent references, even when they may not be as authoritative or original as older references. The reason is that they may afford a better entry into the literature. Of course, many are cited simply because they define new ideas.

The use of the first person plural pronoun does not represent an editorial "we." Rather it reflects the fact that John G. Csernansky, M.D., has joined the preparation of this edition as co-author. John and I have been colleagues for a number of years, and I have the highest respect for both his clinical and research skills. Each of us has contributed to each chapter, so the final product is truly a joint effort. We also wish to thank Lenita Stanley and Pamela J. Elliott for their valuable help in putting together the drafts of each chapter.

We hope this short volume will add information and insight to the reader. If it leads to better treatment of patients, we shall have fulfilled our goal.

*Leo E. Hollister, M.D.*

# Preface to the Second Edition

Second editions of books create problems. What should be repeated from the previous edition and what should be deleted? How many readers of the second edition will have read the first? How to find space to cover the new drugs and new knowledge that have accumulated during the five years between editions? All these decisions must be made in the context of trying to keep the book to the same length as it was before.

My approach to these problems has been to rewrite extensively each of the six chapters of this book. Some have been rewritten more than others, perhaps because the advances in new drugs or new knowledge have been more rapid in one field than in another. Each of the six chapters discusses commonly used types of psychotherapeutic drugs: antianxiety agents, hypnotics, antidepressants, anti-psychotics, and lithium. Although the emphasis is on clinical pharmacology, the latter term is used in a much broader sense than the common present-day usage that makes it equivalent to pharmacokinetics. We are interested in describing the disorders to be treated as well as the very practical matters of what drugs to choose, what doses to use, how long to treat, what may go wrong, and so on. Our idea is to apply pharmacological principles to advance the clinical utility of the drugs in question.

Constraints of time make it impossible to go to press with a totally current book. Sometimes more than a year elapses between the completion of a chapter and the publication of the book. Constraints of space make it impossible to cite every valuable contribution to knowledge about specific drug classes, or to cite every reference that one would like to. One hopes that readers will understand, but that nonetheless the references cited will afford an entry to the literature up to the time of their publication.

Therapeutics, especially in these days of rapid advances, is a changing discipline. One's ideas today may not be the same as they were five years ago. So much the better. One needs to be flexible as new knowledge points to new directions. For the sake of clarity, many controversial issues may be addressed from a single point of view; one hopes that it is right but one can't be positive.

Each chapter of this book is brief enough so that it might be read with reasonable comfort at a single sitting. In addition, the book can be used to look up specific points that may have dropped from one's memory. I hope that the book will be used in both ways.

Many people have contributed to this book, both directly and indirectly. I am especially grateful to my many collaborators who have worked with me in studying these drugs for nearly thirty years. To all who have helped, my heartfelt thanks.

*Leo E. Hollister, M.D.*

# Contents

# 1

## PSYCHOTHERAPEUTIC DRUGS IN THE TREATMENT OF EMOTIONAL DISORDERS

### WHAT IS A MENTAL DISORDER?

The term *mental disorder* seems preferable to *mental illness.* How can one speak of an *illness* or *disease* in the absence of a reasonably firm understanding of pathogenesis or etiology? Even the term *disease* contains a great deal of ambiguity. The most important factor in determining whether or not a condition is considered to be a disease is the importance of the doctor in diagnosis and treatment. In one survey, schizophrenia was considered a *disease* by only 50 percent of secondary school students, but by slightly over 90 percent of general practitioners. Depression was rated even less a disease by only slightly more than 20 percent of secondary school students and 67 percent of general practitioners. Alcoholism, on the other hand, was considered by more of those queried to be a disease than either of the other two. Thus, it is obvious that the concept of disease varies considerably, depending on one's point of view (Campbell et al., 1979).

Assuming that the proper designation is *mental disorder,* how should we define it? One technique is what may be called the "Alice-in-Wonderland" school of semantics: "Words mean what I want them to mean; no more, no less." Thus, one can set up arbitrary definitions of mental disorders, based on a consensual view of experts, as has been done during the past decade with the third edition of the *Diagnostic and Statistical Manual of Mental Disorders* (DSM-III) or its largely unnecessary revision (DSM-IIIR). The advantage of such a system is that one can define rather explicitly the diagnoses being used, even though definitions are tentative and not necessarily congruent with clinical practice.

The disadvantage of such a system is that it is often not universally agreed to; the International Classification of Disease (ICD-10) contains definitions that differ to varying extents from the DSM III and DSM IIIR systems. Furthermore,

1

several sets of independent research diagnostic criteria have been proposed that do not always agree among themselves concerning which patients meet criteria for different disorders (Overall and Hollister, 1979). Nonetheless, the attempt to provide precise definitions of diagnoses is a significant advance over the loose descriptions of the past. The problem of changing descriptions is not peculiar to psychiatric disorders. Medical terminology also changes, perhaps even more rapidly, but such changes are usually due to the discovery of some new pathogen, or a new pathogenetic mechanism, or new gross or microscopic pathology. Alas, these sources of understanding are lacking for mental disorders.

## PREVALENCE OF MENTAL DISORDERS

With the current lack of precision in defining mental disorders, it should not be surprising that the degree of prevalence is not at all certain. The best current estimates are based on the flawed survey of the Epidemiologic Catchment Areas, sponsored by the National Institute of Mental Health (Myers et al., 1984; Robins et al., 1984). This survey was conducted by sampling households in several major urban areas and then conducting interviews of the residents using a diagnostic interview schedule administered by lay interviewers. Estimates were made of the prevalence of mental disorders over a 6-month period and over a lifetime.

The overall 6-month prevalence rate for any mental disorder surveyed varied between 16.8 and 23.4 percent among three principal localities; lifetime prevalence rates varied between 28.8 and 38.0 percent. Anxiety disorders were the most common, the 6-month prevalence varying between 6.6 and 14.9 percent, with lifetime prevalence rates varying between 10.4 and 25.1 percent. Curiously, phobias accounted for most of the anxiety disorders; even the currently fashionable diagnosis of panic disorder was uncommon. Generalized anxiety disorder was not considered to be a possible diagnosis, despite the long-held clinical view that this disorder is the most common anxiety disorder seen by psychiatrists. Somatoform disorders (which formerly might have been called psychophysiologic disorders) were rare, despite the long-held view that these are the most common manifestations of anxiety seen by nonpsychiatric physicians.

Substance abuse disorders were next most frequent, with much less variability in their prevalence. Probably the reduced variability was due to the fact that such disorders are both easier to define and more easily understood by the respondents. Six-month prevalence rates varied between 5.8 and 7.2 percent with lifetime prevalence varying between 15.0 and 18.1 percent. As was expected, dependence on alcohol was most frequent.

Affective disorders classified as depression were somewhat less frequent than might have been anticipated. Even combining major depression and dysthymia, the 6-month prevalence rates varied from 4.3 to 7.0 percent, with lifetime prevalence between 5.8 and 9.9 percent. As was expected, mania was infrequent, with rates ranging from 0.4 to 0.8 percent for 6-months and 0.6 and 1.1 percent for lifetime prevalence.

Schizophrenia was as infrequent as might have been expected, with 6-month rates varying between 0.7 and 1.2 percent (including the few cases with schizophreniform disorders) and 1.1 to 2.0 percent for lifetime prevalence. Severe cognitive impairment, almost exclusively in the age group of 65 years old and over, varied from 1.0 to 1.3 percent.

This monumental effort at trying to estimate the frequency of mental disorders in the general population has provided the best data available, despite its deficiencies. What it suggests is that you only find that for which you ask (no generalized anxiety disorder) and that the more evident the disorder is to the lay public (cognitive disorder, psychosis, alcohol abuse) the smaller the range of variability and the more likely the estimated prevalence rates are accurate.

No matter how one views the statistics, mental disorders affect a sizable number of people. Among the 10 leading causes of death of all age groups, four causes—accidents, suicides, cirrhosis of the liver, and homicide—have strong links with mental disorders (Silverberg and Lubera, 1989). Mortality notwithstanding, morbidity can be very high, as virtually all mental disorders interfere to varying degrees with life functions over long periods of time. At any given moment, almost 2 million people are under some formal treatment for emotional disorders, and psychiatrists now outnumber pediatricians and obstetricians. Most treatment is given by nonpsychiatric physicians, and probably one-half of all visits to family or personal physicians are for treatment of a primary or secondary emotional disorder.

## PSYCHOTHERAPEUTIC DRUGS AND MODERN PSYCHIATRY

Long-term trends may have diminished the importance of mental hospitals, but the advent of effective drugs has hastened the trend almost beyond belief. Mental hospitals that resemble prisons are largely a thing of the past, and for the most part, hospitalized mental patients are encouraged to retain or extend their contacts to the community. Many more patients are discharged into the community; resident population has declined by 80 percent since 1955. Many older mental hospitals have been converted to other uses, and the few new ones being built are generally smaller, closer to academic medical centers, and staffed for a rapid turnover of patients.

Treatment of emotional disorders has been shifted to the community. Some thoughtful observers are concerned that patients are being sent back to the community prematurely, often into totally inadequate surroundings that are reminiscent of the older-type mental hospital. Flourishing community mental health centers have not filled the gap, as they tend to avoid involvement with the most severely ill patients. Thus, an unanticipated adverse effect of the advent of effective drugs is that they not only permitted the release of many long-term mental hospital patients but also spawned the belief that somehow these patients can be maintained in the community with minimal resources. Currently, several hundreds of thousands of homeless persons, wandering the streets of major cities, more properly belong back in mental hospitals.

In addition to the changes in psychiatric practice, a major change in psychiatric thinking has developed during the past 30 years. From 1920 to 1955, psychoanalysis provided the main intellectual foundations of psychiatry. For the past three decades, the emphasis has been on neurobiology, largely as the result of the development of effective drug therapies. Oddly enough, even in the prior epoch, the contributions of biologic psychiatry were considerable. Only three major emotional disorders have been virtually eliminated in this century by effective prevention and treatment: (1) the psychosis associated with niacin deficiency (pellagra), (2) that associated with central nervous system syphilis (dementia paralytica, or general paresis), and (3) the dementia associated with uncontrolled epilepsy. The full extent to which new techniques of imaging the living brain or identifying genes may advance psychiatric understanding and treatment remains to be revealed. However, psychopharmacology has once again reestablished the bridge between psychiatry and biology (Pardes, 1986).

A new model of psychiatrist may emerge. Psychiatrists, because of their medical training, should have an appreciation of both the biologic and psychosocial aspects of people. They may choose to function more or less in one domain or the other. They would be generally informed about all systems but more expert and knowledgeable about particular ones. The present tendency to think that biologic determinants act on the mind differently from social determinants may be too simplistic. What happens to an animal (or human) may permanently change the function of the brain. Many years ago, David Krech showed that animals reared essentially in sensory isolation had smaller brains with less acetylcholine than animals not so reared. More recently, the plasticity of the nervous system in relation to external inputs has been demonstrated for a variety of stimuli. Sensory deprivation and learning have profound biologic consequences, causing effective disruption of synaptic connections under some circumstances, and reactivation of connections under others (Kandel, 1979). Thus, we can no longer embrace a dualistic "either–or" view of the mind.

## NOMENCLATURE OF PSYCHOTHERAPEUTIC DRUGS

The original term for these new drugs, *tranquilizers,* was clearly a poor choice. It created much misunderstanding about the value of psychotherapeutic drugs. Many, opposed on ideologic grounds to all drug therapy of emotional disorders, construed these drugs to be "chemical straitjackets." Much evidence to the contrary has developed over the past two decades, so that these drugs may more properly be called liberating when correctly used.

The term *psychotherapeutic* is difficult to apply to drugs, as it formerly was used exclusively to denote some form of psychological or social, rather than pharmacologic, therapy. The alternate, *psychotropic,* is less precise in its meaning, for it includes many drugs with psychic actions that are not therapeutic. An even more prolific array of terms has been used to describe specific classes of drugs. Drugs used predominantly to treat anxiety have been termed *sedatives, minor tranquilizers, muscle relaxants, psychorelaxants,* and *anxiolytic drugs.* Drugs for treating depression have been called *psychostimulants* (some tricyclic antidepressants clearly are not), *psychic energizers*, or *thymoleptics*. The antischizophrenic drugs were called *major tranquilizers, ataraxics, neuroleptics,* and *psycholeptics*. Because lithium carbonate has proved to be so specific for treating mania whereas so few other drugs are, there has been no hesitancy in referring to it as an *antimanic* drug, although its dual action in preventing depressive episodes as well suggests that more properly it might be considered a *mood stabilizer*. The prefix *anti* has much to recommend it, as it indicates the uses of the various types of drugs. Thus, we may speak of antianxiety drugs, antidepressives, antipsychotics, and antimanic agents.

## TESTING PSYCHOTHERAPEUTIC DRUGS

Controlled clinical trials remain the definitive studies with which to establish the efficacy of a drug, and now are universally required prior to a drug's acceptance for marketing. Large-scale controlled trials are difficult and expensive, and few questions remain that are of sufficient importance to merit the time or expense. Recently, the tendency has been to shift to smaller, controlled trials, with some disadvantages.

The near-total embrace of the controlled clinical trial for proving new drugs has led to some overemphasis on the technique. One now sees controlled trials, often of major magnitude, proposed for a new drug before some of its basic properties are known. Does it have any efficacy at all? What is the proper range of dose? How long is it necessary to treat to show a clear therapeutic response? Should particular patients or symptoms be targeted? What are the common side effects? How close should laboratory monitoring be? The old idea of having three or four experienced clinicians look at the drug in open trials to assess these parameters still has much to commend it.

Recent experience has suggested that although the trials done during the developmental stages of a drug usually confirm its efficacy and safety, the whole story is far from known. The relative efficacy of the drug versus other available agents, its efficacy for particular subgroups of patients, the occurrence of side effects that were missed during the developmental stages or are uncommon, and the efficacy of the drug over the long term often do not come to light until the drug has had extensive use in the actual clinical situation. Accordingly, increasing emphasis is being placed on postmarketing surveillance of drugs to provide answers to some of these vexing questions.

## PRESCRIBING PATTERNS FOR PSYCHOTHERAPEUTIC DRUGS

Physicians are often accused of poor prescribing practices, sometimes with justification, sometimes without. Most concern has centered around the possible overuse of antianxiety and hypnotic drugs and underuse of antidepressants. Most attention has been paid to the patterns of use of anxiolytic drugs. Two surveys of their use in the United States, separated by an interval of almost a decade, showed no evidence for increasing use. In both surveys the drugs were used in an appropriate medical model (Mellinger et al., 1978; Mellinger et al., 1984). More recent surveys from other countries come to similar conclusions. A random sampling of citizens of Munich aged 30 to 69 years showed a 1-week use prevalence of 9.3 percent for all psychotropic drugs. Anxiolytics accounted for two-thirds of the use. The majority of users were women, doses were conservative, drug use tended to increase with increasing age, and both concurrent medical problems or definable stresses were the best predictors of use (Koenig et al., 1987). A similar survey in Belfast found that sedatives and antidepressants were most often prescribed, with hypnotics being used mainly by the elderly. All users tended to be older and to have had a history of physical illness rather than psychosocial problems. In summary, the general practitioners were considered to be discriminating in their prescribing (Irwin and Cupples, 1986). The myth of prescription-happy physicians blithely prescribing psychotherapeutic drugs for trivial indications dies hard.

The proper use of psychotherapeutic drugs is not to be measured by how many people use them, and how often, but under what circumstances and with what effects. The prudent use of psychotherapeutic drugs demands the same skills required for the use of any other type of drug: proper diagnosis, proper selection of drug, proper doses and dosage schedules, and careful clinical follow-up. If these conditions are met, there should be no concern about overuse or underuse. A set of guidelines for peer review has been developed (Dorsey et al., 1979).

## ADVERSE EFFECTS—THE PROBLEMS OF RISK : BENEFIT RATIO

The delayed recognition and appreciation of tardive dyskinesias as a sequel to treatment with antipsychotic drugs has raised many issues with regard to the use of these powerful agents. As a consequence, attempts have been made in varying ways to reduce the total exposure of patients to them. Initial doses for treating patients are lower than those previously used; maintenance treatment either seeks to find a minimum effective dose or to treat on an "as needed" basis. The appearance of early signs of the disorder becomes an indication for discussion about the benefits and risks of continued treatment.

Antidepressant drugs have been plagued by bad luck. Unanticipated adverse reactions ranging from red—green color blindness to multiple peripheral neuropathy to hemolytic anemia have led to the withdrawal of drugs previously marketed and deemed to be both safe and effective. Fortunately, the drugs most widely used have a respectable margin of safety in relation to their efficacy.

Concern about problems of "therapeutic-dose dependence" on benzodiazepines, a complication recognized only during the past decade, has led to a more conservative use of these agents. The number of patients treated with these drugs has not been conspicuously reduced (nor should they be, from all evidence of the frequency of disabling anxiety), but the doses and duration of treatment have been.

Adverse effects are exceedingly difficult to anticipate for individual patients. Thus, risk : benefit ratios are extraordinarily difficult to define. One must simply do one's best for a patient based on existing knowledge.

## THE IDEAL DRUG

The ideal psychotherapeutic drug would (1) act directly on the pathogenetic mechanisms of the symptom or disorder to cure or alleviate it; (2) be effective rapidly; (3) benefit most or all patients for whom it is indicated; (4) be nonhabituating and lack potential for creating dependence; (5) not allow tolerance to develop; (6) have minimum toxicity in the therapeutic range; (7) have a low incidence of secondary side effects; (8) not be lethal in overdoses; (9) be adaptable to both inpatients and outpatients; and (10) not impair any cognitive, perceptual, or motor functions. No such drug exists, but to a fairly surprising degree many of the available drugs meet the majority of these criteria. It has been both a blessing and a curse that we had effective drug therapy for emotional disorders before a science of behavioral pathology. Our best hope now for finding better psychotherapeutic drugs is to understand better the causes and mechanisms of mental disorders.

## REFERENCES

Campbell EJM, Scadding JG, Roberts RS (1979) The concept of disease. Br Med J 2:757–762

Dorsey R, Ayd JF, Jr., Cole J, et al (1979) Psychopharmacological screening criteria development project. JAMA 241:1021–1031

Irwin WG, Cupples ME (1986) A survey of psychotropic drug prescribing. J R Coll Gen Pract 36:366–368

Kandel ER (1979) Psychotherapy and the single synapse: the impact of psychiatric thought on neurobiological research. N Engl J Med 301:1028–1037

Koenig W, Ruther E, Filipiak B (1987) Psychotropic drug utilization patterns in a metropolitan population. Eur J Clin Pharmacol 32:43–51

Mellinger GD, Balter MB, Manheimer DI, et al (1978) Psychic distress, life crisis and use of psychotherapeutic medications: national household survey. Arch Gen Psychiatry 35:1045–1052

Mellinger GC, Balter MB, Uhlenhuth EH (1984) Prevalence and correlates of longterm regular use of anxiolytics. Arch Gen Psychiatry 251:375–379

Myers JK, Weissman MM, Tischler GL, et al (1984) Six-month prevalence of psychiatric disorders in three communities: 1980 to 1982. Arch Gen Psychiatry 41:959–967

Overall JE, Hollister LE (1979) Comparative evaluation of research diagnostic criteria for schizophrenia. Arch Gen Psychiatry 36:1198–1205

Pardes H (1986) Neuroscience and psychiatry: marriage or co-existence? Am J Psychiatry 143:1205–1212

Robins LN, Helzer JE, Weissman MM, et al (1984) Lifetime prevalence of specific psychiatric disorders in three sites. Arch Gen Psychiatry 41:949–958

Silverberg E, Lubera JA (1989) Cancer statistics. CA 39:3–20

# 2

---

# ANTIANXIETY DRUGS

## HISTORY

### Older Drugs

From the time of Greek nepenthe to the present-day use of benzodiazepines, mankind has used sedating drugs to allay the worries of everyday life or the apprehensions of inner anxieties, to promote restful sleep, or to create unconsciousness during painful procedures. For the major portion of the twentieth century, bromides and barbiturates were used as antianxiety drugs. By the 1930s, it had become apparent that the effects of bromides were cumulative and produced a toxic delirium. Chemical assays of plasma bromide concentrations had been developed, but these were used less for monitoring treatment than for diagnosis of toxicity. Misuse of bromides, which were sold freely to the public in pharmacies, finally led to a decline in popularity and their subsequent removal from the market.

Barbiturates were popular sedative–hypnotics during the first half of this century. Short-acting and moderately long-acting drugs, such as secobarbital sodium, amobarbital sodium, and pentobarbital sodium, were used as hypnotics, while the long-acting drug phenobarbital was most commonly employed as an anxiolytic or anticonvulsant. The latter indication for phenobarbital still holds. By the mid-1950s, it was proved that barbiturates produced tolerance and physical dependence. The withdrawal syndrome was similar to that of alcohol. This belated substantiation of a phenomenon clinicians had commonly observed for years made the term *sedative* anathema. The stage was set for the introduction of new agents.

### Newer Drugs

The first of the new drugs was meprobamate, a chemical variant of the weak and very short-acting muscle relaxant mephenesin. The term *tranquilizer* had been coined earlier for chlorpromazine and reserpine. Meprobamate was described as a minor tranquilizer to avoid calling it a sedative, but the term *tranquilizer,* even when qualified as major or minor, was misleading when applied to both classes of drugs. Although initial studies of meprobamate emphasized some differences between it and barbiturates, especially the presumed muscle-relaxant properties, many perceptive pharmacologists quickly recognized that these differences were trivial.

The enormous popularity of meprobamate as the first representative of a group of nonbarbiturate sedatives led to many others. First, the structure of meprobamate itself was manipulated to produce a great variety of similar drugs. Also, modifications of the structure of phenobarbital produced glutethimide, a barbiturate surrogate with no advantages and greater hazards compared to phenobarbital. In general, dissatisfactions with these so-called nonbarbiturates left the demand for different sedative–hypnotics unsatisfied.

During the late 1950s, the drug that ultimately became known as chlordiazepoxide was synthesized. It proved to have remarkable sedative–hypnotic properties in animal pharmacologic testing. Clinical testing confirmed these observations, and the drug was introduced into medical practice in 1960. Since then, an impressive array of other benzodiazepines has been introduced into clinical practice, and new ones continue to appear. Buspirone, a completely novel drug, was introduced in 1987. The place of this drug, and others like it, for treating anxiety remains to be determined.

## Nature of Anxiety

Anxiety is an idiosyncratic symptom. It can be described generally as a pervasive feeling of apprehension that stems from an unknown threat. If the threat is known, the same phenomenon is called fear, and the individual is compelled to take action (either fight or flight). The unknown threat that gives rise to anxiety is often assumed to arise from within the person, in some cases based on a memory of past fear and triggered by unrecognized reminders in the present situation. Such memories may signal the emotions and somatic responses of the past fearful state. The somatic manifestations of anxiety are many, affecting virtually all organ systems. In many cases, the somatic manifestations of anxiety may mimic physical disease, and so must be distinguished from a variety of illnesses that demand medical or surgical therapies. Anxiety and organic disease often have mutually aggravating effects.

Although anxiety is notoriously variable, the recurring sensations felt by individual patients are remarkably consistent. Most of us have had personal experience with the symptom of anxiety, but few have ever experienced the dire sense of foreboding and apprehension that is both discomforting and disabling for many patients. Unlike fear, which is intense but short-lived, anxiety may persist for hours, or days, or years. Because it is a subjective symptom, the degree of anxiety experienced by patients is of lesser importance than its meaning to them. Even though simple anxiety does not often have the potential for serious disability, as do the mood disorders and schizophrenia, it can impair the ordinary functions of human life—love, work, and play. More severe forms of anxiety, such as panic attacks or agoraphobia, may be severely disabling.

# Nosology and Prevalence

In the revised third edition of the *Diagnostic and Statistical Manual for Mental Disorders* published by the American Psychiatric Association a variety of disorders that feature anxiety as a principal symptom are collected under the overall heading Anxiety Disorders. These disorders are summarized in Table 2-1. In many of them, special symptoms that frequently accompany anxiety or represent special forms of anxiety are prominent, such as panic, obsessiveness, and phobias. Interrelationships between anxiety and these other symptoms may well develop as the result of inadvertent conditioning. For example, spontaneous panic attacks may lead to the appearance of anticipatory anxiety and phobic avoidance related to situations in which the panic attacks have occurred. Biologic mechanisms that derive from genetic substrates are now increasingly thought to underlie these disorders, rather than unconscious conflicts. Furthermore, anxiety is often a prominent symptom of many disorders that are not specifically classified as anxiety disorders by DSM-IIIR. For example, anxiety is frequently a concomitant of depression and may be the predominant symptom during the early stages of psychotic decompensation in schizophrenic patients. Many character disorders, in particular those distinguished by primitive interpersonal interactions, also have severe anxiety as a prominent feature. These disorders are also summarized in Table 2-1.

The best and most recent data regarding the relative prevalence of anxiety disorders among various psychiatric disorders was derived from large samples of persons interviewed in several major U.S. cities. One can never be entirely certain about the representativeness of the samples nor of the sensitivity of the interviewing techniques. Still, anxiety disorders were found to be extremely frequent.

The total percentages of interviewees that had anxiety disorders during the past 6-month period ranged from 6.6 to 14.9 percent. Only four subclasses of anxiety disorders were distinguished: phobia, panic, obsessive-compulsive, and somatization. This classification seems strange, considering that for many years generalized anxiety disorder was considered by most clinicians to

## Table 2-1. Anxiety Disorders

Anxiety Disorders Defined by DSM-IIIR
    Generalized anxiety disorder
    Panic disorders with or without agoraphobia
    Social phobia
    Simple phobia
    Obsessive-compulsive disorder
    Post-traumatic stress disorder

Other Major Disorders with Prominent Anxiety
    Major depression
    Schizophrenia
    Dementia
    Adjustment disorder
    Personality disorders, especially "borderline"

be most frequent. Phobias were most frequent, ranging from 5.4 to 13.4 percent, obsessive-compulsive disorder was next, ranging from 1.3 to 2.0 percent. Oddly, somatization, which constitutes such a large amount of medical practice, was rarely found (0.1 percent); panic disorder, a fad diagnosis these days, was also uncommon (0.6 to 1.0 percent). Overall, the 6-month prevalence data indicated that anxiety disorders were the most frequent psychiatric problem (Myers et al., 1984).

As might be expected, lifetime prevalence figures were higher, ranging from 10.4 to 25.1 percent for all anxiety disorders. The same order held for the subgroups, being highest for phobias (7.8 to 23.3 percent), followed by obsessive-compulsive disorder (1.9 to 3.0 percent), panic (1.4 to 1.5 percent) and somatization (0.1 percent). In terms of lifetime prevalence, only substance-abuse disorders outranked anxiety disorders (Robins et al., 1984).

Even though these estimates may be flawed, they indicate that anxiety is very common in the general population. It is little wonder that drugs for treating anxiety find such a ready market.

## Pathogenesis

The sympathomimetic model of fear and anxiety, which traces its roots to Walter Cannon, still provides the most fruitful line of investigation in our attempt to understand the biologic pathogenesis of anxiety. The physiologic changes of anxiety can be induced by a variety of sympathomimetic agents, although it is less sure that the psychological changes are typical of anxiety. For several years, a great deal of attention has been paid to the locus coeruleus, the blue streak at the base of the fourth ventricle, as a site for the production of anxiety. Most of the norepinephrine innervation of the brain originates in neurons located in this nucleus.

Evidence for the involvement of the locus coeruleus in anxiety, at least in humans, is circumstantial. Electrical stimulation of the nucleus in awake monkeys elicits behavior that is associated with fear in the wild. Conversely, lesions of the nucleus prevent fearful behavior in situations where such behavior is the expected response. The firing rate of locus coeruleus neurons is controlled by several neurotransmitter systems, giving support to the notion that there may exist several approaches to anxiolysis. Neurotransmitter systems that affect the locus coeruleus include serotonin, acetylcholine, GABA, and several neuropeptides, in addition to alpha-2 adrenergic autoreceptors on the cell body. Drugs that increase the firing of neurons in the nucleus, such as piperoxan and yohimbine, elicit some symptoms of anxiety, whereas drugs that decrease firing, such as clonidine, barbiturates, and benzodiazepines, tend to reduce anxiety. Interestingly, a new anxiolytic drug, buspirone, appears to be an exception to this rule, as it increases locus coeruleus firing (Sanghera et al., 1983). Blockade of the postsynaptic effects of norepinephrine by beta-adrenoreceptor blocking drugs also tends to mitigate anxiety (Mason and Fibiger, 1979).

It would seem reasonable that one might test these notions in humans. Pharmacologically induced models of anxiety in humans would be most useful, not only to further explore the pathogenesis of anxiety but also to test new potential therapeutic agents. Recent work by Charney and Heninger (1986a) has suggested that there may be increased sensitivity to both alpha-2 adrenergic agonists and antagonists in patients with panic disorder. Furthermore, they have demonstrated that at least two of the presynaptic influences on the locus coeruleus, the opioid system and alpha-2 autoreceptors have convergent effects in modulating anxiety (Charney and Heninger, 1986b).

## CHEMICAL CLASSES OF ANTIANXIETY DRUGS

The dominance of the benzodiazepines in clinical practice is all the more remarkable because of the many types of agents that can be used for, and have been promoted for, the treatment of anxiety. At least seven different chemical classes of such drugs can be described (Table 2-2). One group, exemplified by barbiturates, meprobamate and its congeners, and benzodiazepines, has the classic profile of pharmacologic actions that identify these drugs as *sedative–hypnotics:* sedation proceeding to hypnosis, muscle relaxation, and anticonvulsant action. Unfortunately, this group is well known for producing tolerance as well as psychological and physical dependence.

A second group of antianxiety agents can be termed *sedative–autonomic,* for lack of a better term. This term indicates that they differ from the sedative–hypnotics in having variable effects on the peripheral autonomic nervous system, via anticholinergic or anti-alpha-adrenergic actions. In addition, the sedation these drugs produce is qualitatively different from that of the sedative–hypnotics. Sedative–autonomic drugs include various antihistamines, some of which are sold without prescription as sedatives or hypnotics, antipsychotic drugs in small doses, and some of the more sedative tricyclic antidepressants. These drugs also differ from the sedative–hypnotic group in that they increase muscle tone and lower the convulsive threshold. They have a minimal predisposition for producing tolerance or dependence. However, patients find the qualitatively different sedation and autonomic side effects of sedative–autonomic drugs unpleasant. In fact, the same reasons that make these drugs less likely to be abused by patients also make them less likely to be accepted.

**Table 2-2.  Classes of Antianxiety Drugs**

Sedative–hypnotic
    Barbiturates: phenobarbital
    Nonbarbiturates: meprobamate
    Benzodiazepines: diazepam

Sedative–autonomic
    Antihistamines: diphenhydramine
    Antidepressants: doxepin
    Antipsychotics: trifluoperazine

Other
    Azaspirodecanediones: buspirone

Buspirone represents a novel antianxiety drug, an azaspirodecanedione. It has been widely promoted for its lack of abuse potential. This drug has neither overt sedative, hypnotic, or autonomic actions and is unlike almost all other drugs used to treat anxiety. Drugs of this class could become strong competitors with the popular benzodiazepines.

## Chemical Modifications of the Benzodiazepine Nucleus

A great number of benzodiazepines with anxiolytic activity are possible on the basis of chemical variation. The basic benzodiazepine nucleus has been substituted at six different positions to produce compounds with varying degrees of pharmacologic potency and routes of metabolism, as shown in Figure 2-1.

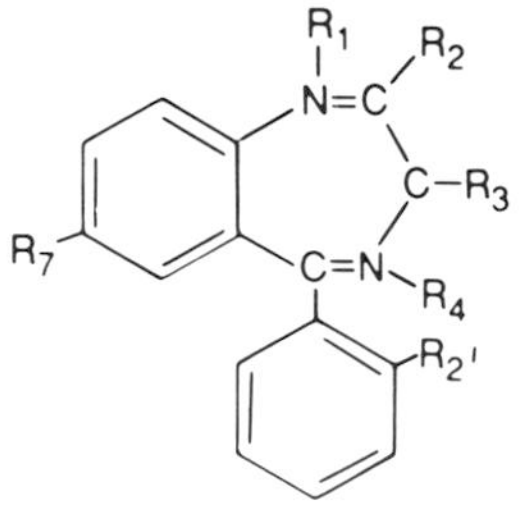

Benzodiazepine nucleus and points of chemical substitutions

alprazolam

$R_2$= =N-N-CH(CH$_3$)·R$_1$;R$_2$=Cl

chlordiazipoxide

$R_2$=NCH$_3$;R$_7$=Cl

clonazepam

$R_2$=O;R$_2^1$=Cl;R$_7$=NO$_2$

clorazepate

$R_2$=OH,O⁻;R$_3$=COO⁻;R$_7$=Cl

diazepam

$R_1$=CH$_3$;R$_2$=O;R$_7$=Cl

halazepam

$R_1$=CH$_2$CF$_3$;R$_2$=O;R$_7$=Cl

lorazepam

$R_2$=O;R$_3$=OH;R$_7$=Cl;R$_2^1$=Cl

midazolam

$R_1R_2$ =

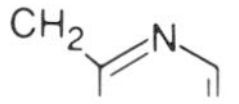

$R_7$ = Cl

$R_2'$ = F

oxazepam

$R_3$=OH;R$_7$=Cl

prazepam

$R_1$ = CH$_2$-CH$_2$-CH$_2$; R$_2$ = = O ; R$_7$ = Cl
CH$_2$

**Fig. 2-1.** Structural relationships of various antianxiety benzodiazepines. Differences in pharmacokinetic aspects are more evident than pharmacodynamic actions. The uses for which drugs are promoted often have little bearing on either.

Whether or not the spectrum of pharmacologic activity varies as much is still an unsettled question. Nonetheless, several of these drugs have been promoted for different indications on the basis of such changes. For instance, flurazepam and temazepam are promoted only as hypnotics, clonazepam only as an anticonvulsant, diazepam as an antianxiety drug, muscle relaxant, anticonvulsant, and anesthetic, and midazolam solely as an anesthetic.

## Mechanism of Benzodiazepine Action

The discovery by two laboratories in 1977 of specific receptors for benzodiazepines in the brains of various mammals triggered a tremendous amount of investigation into the modes of action of these drugs and gave strong support to the hypothesis that some forms of anxiety may have a biologic basis (Squires and Braestrup, 1977; Mohler and Okada, 1977). The clinical potency of the benzodiazepines as anxiolytics parallels their affinity for these receptors. Subsequent investigations proved that benzodiazepine receptors are functionally linked to one of the two subtypes of gamma-aminobutyric acid receptors (GABA-A), and that together these two receptors regulate the opening and closing of a chloride ion channel (see Figure 2-2). Both GABA and the benzodiazepines act to enhance the capacity of each other to open the chloride channel and hyperpolarize the postsynaptic cell (Tallman et al., 1980).

Specific antagonists of the benzodiazepines, such as flumazenil, also block the physiologic actions of GABA and GABA agonists (Mohler and Richards, 1981). Such drugs may find clinical utility as treatments for benzodiazepine overdose.

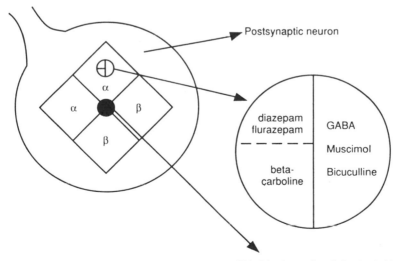

**Fig. 2-2.** Representation of the GABA/benzodiazepine receptor complex. The protein is a tetramere composed of two alpha and two beta subunits. The GABA and benzodiazepine receptors are most likely located on the alpha subunits. Benzodiazepine receptors may bind agonists, antagonists (flumazenil), or inverse agonists (beta-carboline).

Other drugs, such as picrotoxin, can directly bind to the chloride channel to block chloride ion flow. Furthermore, activation of this picrotoxin site also modulates the function of GABA and the benzodiazepines at their respective receptors. Nonbenzodiazepine anxiolytics, such as the barbiturates, compete with picrotoxin for binding to this site, thereby directly increasing ion flow as well as enhancing GABA and benzodiazepine-mediated events (Skolnick and Moncada, 1981).

A third type of ligand that binds to benzodiazepine receptors is exemplified by some beta-carbolines and an endogenous peptide, diazepam-binding inhibitor (DBI). DBI is a polypeptide with a molecular weight of 10,000 daltons that inhibits benzodiazepine binding and blocks the actions of GABA (Alho et al., 1985). More recently, several smaller fragments of this peptide have also been identified in brain and have been shown to have anxiogenic actions in animals. Substances such as these may be viewed as "inverse agonists," in the sense that they produce an action contrary to the benzodiazepines. It is possible that the benzodiazepine receptor exists in different functional states, each one referring to activation by ligands with differing action (Martin, 1987; Costa, 1988).

Studies of the benzodiazepine receptor may also shed light on a biologic mechanism for the production of anxiety. The normal function of the benzodiazepine receptor might be to provide a basis for the development of anxiety or fear, an important defense mechanism, mediated through some endogenous ligand such as DBI. Symptoms may occur when the function of the benzodiazepine receptor complex becomes disturbed as the result of some inborn abnormality or an environmental stimulation early in life that leads to exaggerated responses to stress throughout life. Thus, we may have an explanation for the subpopulation of persons who have chronic pathologic anxiety and seem to benefit from antianxiety drugs (Haefely, 1985).

## METABOLISM AND KINETICS OF BENZODIAZEPINES
### Metabolism

Dealkylation, oxidation, reduction, and glucuronidation are the principal metabolic pathways of the various benzodiazepines. Several routes may be employed with some compounds, producing a succession of active metabolites. Some of the metabolic interrelationships between various commonly used benzodiazepines are shown in Figure 2-3. Chlordiazepoxide, for instance, first undergoes dealkylation, then oxidation and reduction to form a common metabolite of many of these agents, N-desmethyldiazepam (nordiazepam).

Most benzodiazepines are extensively metabolized. The central position of nordiazepam in the metabolism has been depicted in Figure 2-3. On the other hand, drugs with a free hydroxyl group, such as oxazepam and lorazepam, readily form glucuronides, which can be excreted without further metabolism. As metabolism of drugs is definitely impaired in patients with liver disease, and may be impaired in elderly patients, oxazepam and lorazepam have been suggested as the drugs of choice in these two situations.

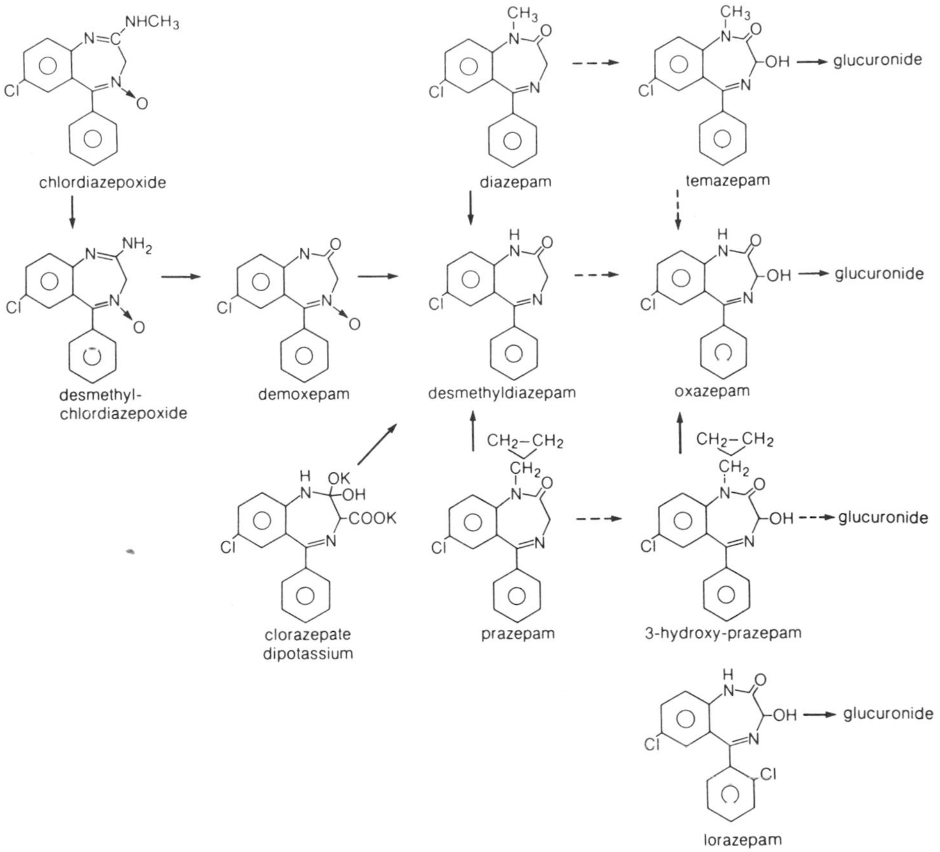

**Fig. 2-3.** Metabolic pathways for various types of benzodiazepines. The central position of *N*-desmethyldiazepam (nordiazepam) is evident.

Some drugs on the market are essentially prodrugs for nordiazepam, being very quickly converted from the parent compound to their active metabolite. This may occur either by dealkylation, as in the case of prazepam, or by hydrolysis, as in the case of clorazepate dipotassium. Drugs that have a hydroxyl group at the 3 position form no active metabolites but are directly conjugated.

## Kinetics

The pharmacokinetic parameters of various benzodiazepines are summarized in Table 2-3. A number of reviews of the pharmacokinetics of these drugs have appeared recently (Greenblatt and Shader, 1985; Williams et al., 1985; Ellinwood et al., 1985; Saletu and Pakesch, 1987).

The major differences between the various members are in relation to plasma half-life and degree of metabolism. Based on plasma half-life, drugs have been classified as very short-, short-, intermediate-, long- and very long-acting

## Table 2-3. Pharmacokinetic Parameters of Antianxiety Benzodiazepines

| Drug | T1/2b (h) | VD (L/Kg) | Protein Binding | Active Metabolites | T1/2b (h) | Therapeutic Concentration (ng/ml) |
|---|---|---|---|---|---|---|
| Very Short | | | | | | |
| Midazolam | 1.5–2.5 | | | 1-Methylhydroxy | | |
| Short | | | | | | |
| Alprazolam | 6–20 | 0.7–0.8 | | | | |
| Lorazepam | 9–22 | 0.7–1.0 | 85 | None | | |
| Oxazepam | 6–24 | 0.6–1.6 | 86 | None | | |
| Intermediate | | | | | | |
| Chlordiazepoxide | 10–29 | 0.3–0.6 | 93 | Desmethyl | 10–18 | |
| | | | | Desmoxepam | 28–63 | |
| | | | | Desoxydemoxepam | 39–61 | |
| Clonazepam | 19–42 | | | | | |
| Diazepam | 14–61 | 0.7–2.6 | 98 | Nordiazepam | 36–200 | 400–1200 |
| Halazepam | 9–28 | 0.1–1.3 | 98 | Nordiazepam | 36–200 | |
| Long | | | | | | |
| Clorazepate | | 1.0–1.3 | 98 | Nordiazepam | 36–200 | 430 |
| Prazepam | | 1.0–1.3 | 98 | Nordiazepam | 36–200 | 430 |

compounds. However, the actual duration of action of these drugs may vary slightly from such a classification, based on metabolites with longer actions.

Virtually all benzodiazepines are highly lipophilic, a characteristic that allows nearly complete absorption after oral administration with rapid penetration into the brain. Midazolam and diazepam are the most lipophilic compounds. Some, such as lorazepam and midazolam are water-soluble, which allows them to be used either intramuscularly or intravenously with more safety and convenience. Other compounds, such as chlordiazepoxide and diazepam, are not readily available when given intramuscularly.

Lipid solubility also ensures that most of these drugs have relatively large apparent volumes of distribution. Almost all have dual-phase plasma half-lives, the more rapid initial phase being largely due to distribution and the slower, later phase being due to metabolic elimination. In the case of highly lipid soluble drugs, such as diazepam, termination of the clinical effects of single doses of the drug is mainly due to extensive distribution to the lipid components of the body.

Protein-binding of these drugs is generally high. Because of the great amount of drug sequestered in the body as a result of high protein-binding and distribution to tissues, the amount of drug available for dialysis is small; overdoses are not treated with this attempt to eliminate the drug.

Attempts to relate plasma concentrations of these drugs to their acute clinical effects have not been very successful. What is most readily measurable clinically are the effects of sedation. Animal studies indicate that tolerance to this effect may develop quickly, even with single doses (Henauer et al., 1984). Thus, impairment is usually noted as the plasma concentrations are rising but clears when they are falling. A clockwise hysteresis curve relating plasma concentrations to clinical effect therefore ensues. Such a curve is thought to represent single-dose tolerance.

It has been equally difficult to define a range of steady-state therapeutic plasma concentrations of these drugs. Following 14 days of treatment with diazepam, plasma concentrations of nordiazepam were related to dose, but no significant association between clinical symptoms of anxiety and serum diazepam and nordiazepam levels was noted (Tyrer et al., 1984). Thus, although measurements of plasma concentrations can be made readily, no one has ever proposed using them to monitor clinical effects. The clinical response to the drug is more than adequate to define the doses required.

As only the free fraction of any drug is pharmacologically active, the high degree of protein-binding of benzodiazepines indicates that this fraction will be small. If the concentrations of drug in cerebrospinal fluid is considered to represent the free fraction, then only a small fraction of the drug in the body has access to the brain. It is known that different members of this class have different affinities for the benzodiazepine receptor, and variations in affinity may affect duration of action. Lorazepam has been suggested to have a greater affinity for receptors than other drugs and consequently a longer span of clinical effects than indicated by the plasma half-life (Colburn and Jack, 1987).

The chronopharmacology of benzodiazepines has scarcely been investigated. Changes in rate of metabolism over time may be possible, although such changes have not been demonstrated for lorazepam. In monkeys, reduced metabolism of clonazepam was associated with periods of physical inactivity. Diurnal variations have been noted in the responses to midazolam, protein binding of diazepam, and rate of absorption of several of these drugs (Guentert, 1984). Such variations may account for the experience of investigators that plasma concentrations of these drugs often are erratic rather than following smooth rates of decline. Whether or not such variations are of any clinical importance, given the wide range of plasma concentrations achieved from any dosing schedule, is open to question.

## Pharmacokinetic Differences and Clinical Use

As the pharmacodynamic actions of various benzodiazepines may be little different, differences in pharmacokinetics may suggest specific indications for certain compounds. The rapid onset of action when diazepam is given orally, as well as its long duration of action through its major metabolite, nordiazepam, may account for its immense popularity. Absorption is slower with several other drugs. Both diazepam and lorazepam can be given intravenously, unlike some other drugs, which makes them especially valuable for the acute treatment of epilepsy or alcohol withdrawal reactions. Midazolam has been used intravenously for treating very anxious patients, but such use must be done with exceeding care. Lorazepam is suitable for intramuscular administration and has been used with benefit for calming excited, usually psychotic, patients.

Why chlordiazepoxide is less preferred by patients than diazepam or some other drugs, such as lorazepam, is not clear. Like diazepam, it has a long span of action, mediated by the formation of long-lived metabolites.

Drugs with a shorter span of action, such as oxazepam, lorazepam, and alprazolam, have been suggested as being especially useful for treating elderly patients or those with liver disease. Although it is true that these are both situations in which drug elimination can be impaired, the problem may also be dealt with by decreasing the initial dose of drug and by increasing the dosing interval. Thus, longer-acting drugs could be used equally well, with perhaps less drug being needed. Short-acting drugs present problems when once-daily administration is desired.

Drugs that are merely prodrugs for nordiazepam, such as clorazepate dipotassium and prazepam, offer no advantage over diazepam. The latter drug not only provides a substantial amount of nordiazepam, but also the virtues of the parent drug. The latter is presumed to provide sedation. If sedation is a serious problem with diazepam, then nordiazepam prodrugs might be advantageous.

## GENERAL CONSIDERATIONS OF CLINICAL USE

Use of antianxiety drugs increased rapidly following the introduction of the first benzodiazepines in the early 1960s. The rapidly rising rate of prescriptions peaked in the mid-1970s, and since then has declined about 25 percent (Fig.

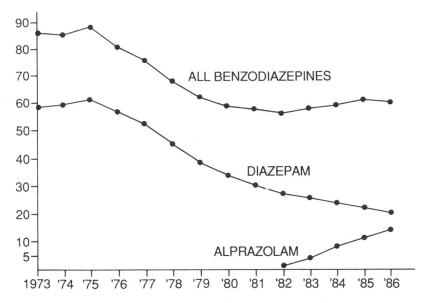

**Fig. 2-4.** Total prescriptions in the United States, minor tranquilizers–benzodiazepines. (Data from IMS America Ltd. National Prescription Audit, 1987.)

2-4). The declining use stemmed largely from fears about possible dependence on benzodiazepines. Since the early 1980s, use of short-acting, more potent benzodiazepines, such as lorazepam and alprazolam, has increased at the expense of older compounds, such as diazepam.

Antianxiety drugs continue to be controversial. Many believe that to rely on drug therapy for the treatment of symptoms rooted in life experience may deny patients the benefits of other treatments, particularly psychotherapy, which may be more specific and permanent. Although the efficacy of these drugs for relieving the symptoms of anxiety is generally accepted, many doubt that the patients who take them are benefited overall. Finally, the rapid increase in nonmedical use of mind-altering drugs has led to concerns that overenthusiastic prescribing of these drugs may contribute to this problem.

Concerns about the rapid increase in use of benzodiazepines led the National Institute of Mental Health in the early 1970s to commission a large epidemiologic study of their use. Findings were reassuring. Only 9.6 to 16.8 percent of interviewees in 10 different countries had used any of these drugs within the preceding year (15 percent in the United States). In terms of continued use for 1 month or more, the range was 3.4 to 8.6 percent (6 percent in the United States). Furthermore, most respondents obtained "substantial benefit" (Balter et al., 1974).

Further analysis of the data from this survey indicated that physicians prescribe these drugs using a typical medical model, the rate of prescription increasing proportional to the degree of "life stress" or "psychic distress" reported by the patients (Mellinger et al., 1978). The actual number of persons with high levels of stress was considerably greater than the number who took drugs, indicating that many persons were able to cope with stress without the use of drugs at all.

A similar survey in 1979 found that regular daily use for 1 year or longer was only the case in 15 percent of people who used these drugs at all, representing only 1.6 percent of adults in the United States. Most users were women, most had sought medical help from mental health professionals, and most were being adequately supervised by their physicians (Mellinger et al., 1984).

The conclusion drawn from these surveys was that these drugs were not being used in a capricious or casual fashion, but rather in a true medical model.

# INDICATIONS

## Anxiety

Feelings of nervousness or constant worry of uncertain cause are a prime indication for the antianxiety drugs. They are especially valuable when symptoms are severe, rather than when they are mild, and when agitation is present. Concomitant symptoms of depression are not a contraindication, but should alert the physician to the possibility that depression is the patient's primary diagnosis. Failure to respond to an antianxiety drug and the new appearance of depression during treatment makes this possibility more likely. As anxiety is a nonspecific symptom, it may also be an early sign of other serious emotional disorders, such as schizophrenia. Again, failure to respond should alert one to diagnostic reconsideration. Usually, given the proper dose of drugs, one would expect to see some positive response within the first week of treatment, even though optimal effects may not be obtained for up to 3 weeks.

Numerous controlled clinical trials have found various benzodiazepines superior to placebo for treatment of anxiety. Although a few studies have been unable to distinguish the two, the chances of negative bias are great in such studies, so considerably more weight must be attached to those studies that show the drug to be superior (Bellantuono et al., 1980).

A number of syndromes are now included under the general rubric of anxiety disorders (Table 2-1). Such a classification merely represents the thinking of some experts at a particular period of history. It is not immutable and could be proven wrong by later developments.

### Generalized Anxiety Disorder

Patients with generalized anxiety disorder (GAD) were diagnosed as having "anxiety reactions" or "anxiety neurosis" in earlier classifications. Persons with this form of free-floating anxiety probably constitute the category of patients most often seen by physicians. Drugs and/or psychotherapy have traditionally been used in generalized anxiety. Although some proponents of psychotherapy insist that drugs impair the treatment of GAD, most evidence suggests that the two modalities work additively.

Although benzodiazepines have long been the preferred drugs for treating GAD, a new class of drugs, exemplified by buspirone, has aroused a great deal of interest. Buspirone is chemically and pharmacologically different from the benzodiazepines. The chemical structure is somewhat reminiscent of the butyro-phenones (Fig. 2-5). It does not act on the benzodiazepine-GABA receptor, but rather at the 5-HT$_{1A}$ serotonin receptor. Such an approach to treating anxiety was previously unknown. In addition, it is a weak antagonist at the D$_2$ do-pamine receptor, which initially led to its consideration as an antipsychotic drug (Taylor, 1988). Although completely absorbed, its systemic bioavailability is low (about 4 percent) because of a great first-pass metabolism. As is true of many psychoactive drugs, it has a large apparent volume of distribution (5.3 L/kg) and a high degree of protein binding (95 percent). Metabolites may be active. The plasma half-life is very short, in the range of 2 to 8 hours.

Most clinical trials of the drug have found it to be more effective than placebo and equivalent to benzodiazepines. A peculiar aspect of its action is that

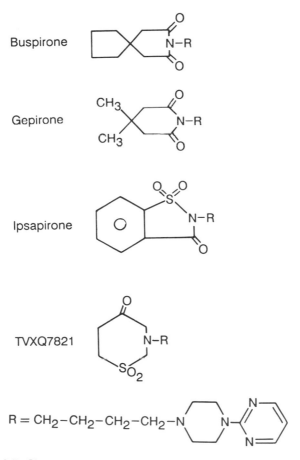

**Fig. 2-5.** Chemical structure of buspirone and related compounds.

improvement is delayed by 2 or 3 weeks, leading some patients and clinicians to doubt its efficacy (Olajida and Lader, 1987; Pecknold et al., 1985). In fact, the drug is poorly accepted by GAD patients who had previously been treated with benzodiazepines. Those who have had such treatment should not be abruptly discontinued from the benzodiazepine lest symptoms become worse, because of either rebound or withdrawal. This lack of cross-tolerance with other sedatives or alcohol makes buspirone inappropriate for treating alcohol withdrawal syndromes.

The major advantage of the drug is that it produces no overt sedation, seemingly having realized the Holy Grail of separating anxiolytic from sedative effects. Thus, functions during waking hours are unimpaired. Neither is there any additive sedative effect with alcohol or other sedative drugs. Finally, lack of sedative effects makes buspirone unattractive as a drug of abuse and no withdrawal reactions have been observed (Lader, 1987).

Buspirone might best be considered as a potential treatment for patients with GAD who have not previously been treated with benzodiazepines. It might also be a suitable alternative for patients with a history of drug abuse, including alcohol, once the patients have been withdrawn from their previous drug of abuse (Palmer, 1988).

Which benzodiazepine to use when treating GAD is a highly subjective matter. It would be manifestly impossible for any clinician to be able to use all the available benzodiazepines. To remember only the generic and trade names would be difficult even for an expert in the field. When faced with a variety of drugs having similar actions, it is far better to learn to use a few well rather than to use all of them poorly. Yet, as mentioned earlier, the bases for selection of benzodiazepines are flimsy, relying more on pharmacokinetic than pharmaco-dynamic differences. Thus, any advice about winnowing down the group is likely to be contentious.

If patients have been previously treated with a benzodiazepine, the logical course would be to re-treat with whichever drug was best tolerated and most effective for them. However, a reasonable selection of benzodiazepines might include a short-, intermediate-, and long-acting drug. Lorazepam or alprazolam would be reasonable choices for a short-acting drug. For the intermediate-acting selection, diazepam is the logical choice. The enormous popularity of this benzodiazepine relative to the others is difficult to explain, but it is preferred by most patients over virtually all others. For the long-acting selection, clorazepate dipotassium would be reasonable. Any of the other prodrugs for nordiazepam might have been chosen, but these drugs have to rely on the whims of metabolism to become active whereas clorazepate needs only to be hydrolyzed. It would not be a suitable drug for those rare patients with little or no stomach acid (Hollister, 1984).

## Panic Disorders

States resembling acute fear, with sudden attacks of breathlessness, tachycardia, trembling, sweating, and a feeling of impending doom, have been known for many years. Variants of this theme have been called "neurocirculatory asthenia," as well as many other names. Until the 1970s most clinicians considered them to be merely acute anxiety attacks in the context of generalized, chronic anxiety. Because panic disorder has been considered a separate entity, the diagnosis is made with increasing frequency. Some cases exist without much generalized anxiety, although most develop some degree of "anticipatory anxiety." Others may be associated with phobias, especially agoraphobia, or with depression. The relationship between panic attacks and these other syndromes is presently unclear.

Imipramine was first reported to be effective in blocking panic attacks in the mid-1960s. Although the efficacy of other tricyclic antidepressants in blocking panic attacks has not been systematically studied, all tricyclic antidepressants are thought to have this effect. Imipramine can be effectively combined with supportive or behavioral psychotherapy in the treatment of panic attacks, but it may also be used to advantage as the sole treatment (Garakani et al., 1984).

Monoamine oxidase inhibitors, such as phenelzine, have also been demonstrated to be effective in the treatment of panic attacks. A double-blind comparison of imipramine, phenelzine, and placebo in 57 patients with panic attacks found phenelzine, 45 mg/day, to be as effective as or slightly superior to imipramine, 150 mg/day. Both drugs were superior to placebo (Sheehan et al., 1980).

Alprazolam, a triazolobenzodiazepine with potential antidepressant as well as antianxiety effects, was found in a multicenter double-blind placebo-controlled study to be effective in blocking panic attacks and associated phobic avoidance (Ballenger et al., 1988). Whether alprazolam is unique among benzodiazepines in its antipanic action has been increasingly questioned. A double-blind study involving 21 patients has shown that diazepam may be effective when used alone as a treatment for panic disorder (Noyes et al., 1984). Other studies have indicated efficacy for clonazepam and lorazepam. As might be expected, larger doses than usual are needed to control this more severe manifestation of anxiety.

## Agoraphobia

Fear of public places is the most common phobia. Many of these patients become completely house-bound. Formerly, the disorder was thought to be of psychic origin, but traditional psychotherapy has generally been ineffective. Behavioral treatments aimed at desensitizing the fear have been more successful, often used concomitantly with monoamine oxidase inhibitors, tricyclic antidepressants, or benzodiazepines.

## Agoraphobia with Panic Attacks

An association between agoraphobia and panic attacks is being recognized with increasing frequency. The issue of which is primary is still unsettled. The older view was that panic ensued when the fearful stimulus could not be avoided. A currently popular view is precisely opposite, that is, the occurrence of a panic attack in a public place leads to the phobia in an effort to avoid future attacks. Theoretical issues aside, it is fortunate that both disorders can be treated with drugs that are used to treat panic disorders alone.

## Social Phobias

Fear of the scrutiny of others is less common than agoraphobia. This disorder is often associated with generalized anxiety, which can be treated as above. Psychotherapies of various kinds have also been tried.

## Specific Phobias

Fears of specific stimuli, such as snakes, dogs, mice, or insects, are relatively uncommon as clinical syndromes requiring treatment. Avoidance of the stimulus or desensitization through behavioral techniques are the most commonly used treatments.

## Obsessive-Compulsive Disorders

Intrusive thoughts, often of danger to self or to others, or a subjective urge to repeat meaningless rituals, often washing of hands, characterize obsessive-compulsive disorder. About 20 percent of patients have family members with the same disorder. Currently it is believed that the disorder represents some sort of dysfunction of the basal ganglia. Neurosurgical approaches to treatment are sometimes a last resort. Behavioral therapy is effective, especially for rituals. The tricyclic antidepressant clomipramine seems to be specifically effective for this disorder, more so than other tricyclics. As clomipramine (but not its metabolite, desmethylclomipramine) specifically blocks uptake of serotonin, a serotonin hypothesis for obsessive-compulsive disorder has been formulated. Many other specific uptake inhibitors of serotonin are currently under investigation for the treatment of this disorder (Rapoport, 1988).

# Hypnosis

The use of benzodiazepines and other drugs for hypnosis will be discussed in Chapter 3.

# Muscle Spasm

Diazepam has been widely used for treating muscle spasm associated with disseminated sclerosis, tetanus, cerebral palsy, and stroke. Debate still exists about the concept of a centrally acting muscle relaxant, because muscle relaxation could occur secondary to sedation. Yet diazepam could have a specific action related to its GABA-enhancing effects. GABA is known to decrease the firing rate of motor neurons in the spinal cord via presynaptic inhibition.

The use of antianxiety drugs, including meprobamate-like compounds such as methocarbamol, for treating simple muscle strains should be discouraged. Judicious use of local physical measures and adequate doses of aspirin are more to the point.

# Uncontrolled, Repeated Seizures

Diazepam given intravenously has long been the drug of choice for the treatment of status epilepticus. Because of rapid entry of the drug into the brain, control is readily attained. However, sustained control requires a subsequent loading dose of phenytoin. Some benzodiazepines, such as clonazepam and clorazepate dipotassium, have been promoted for limited use in convulsive disorders. At least one comparison between clorazepate dipotassium and phenobarbital for maintenance treatment of epilepsy showed that patients preferred the former drug (Wilensky et al., 1981).

## Alcohol Withdrawal

Alcohol withdrawal is best treated with benzodiazepines because: (1) they have pharmacologic properties that are similar to alcohol; (2) they are effective anticonvulsants, affording protection against this frequent complication of alcohol withdrawal; (3) they are not harmful, as phenothiazines, sedative antihistaminics, or barbiturates can be; and (4) they are not noxious, as is paraldehyde. Paraldehyde was compared with diazepam in treating patients with severe delirium tremens (Thompson et al., 1975). Giving diazepam in initial doses of 10 mg intravenously followed by 5 mg every 5 minutes until the patients were calm yet awake was rapidly effective. Maintenance doses were given intramuscularly in this study; however, it is preferable to give them orally unless contraindicated. In milder cases of alcohol withdrawal, oral doses of diazepam can be used entirely.

## Intravenous Anesthesia

Diazepam and lorazepam have been used as intravenous anesthetics. Sufficient anesthesia may be obtained from these drugs alone for brief operative procedures such as electric cardioversion, endoscopic procedures, dental surgery, and reductions of minor fractures. Both have also been used orally as preoperative medications and were superior to barbiturate for this purpose (Wilson and Ellis, 1973). Lorazepam may produce more anterograde amnesia than diazepam. Midazolam has become the preferred intravenously used benzodiazepine anesthetic.

## Special Forms of Anxiety and Agitation

The use of benzodiazepines is now being touted for the treatment of acute mania. Although one might invoke the anticonvulsant properties of the benzodiazepines to explain such antimanic effects, their benefit might be more simply explained by their sedative properties. Although particular compounds, such as lorazepam and clonazepam, have been associated with these claims, few controlled comparisons have been made. Certainly, many drugs with sedative effects should have an important adjunctive role in mitigating the acute agitation and sometimes severe anxiety that occurs in mania and other psychoses. For too long we have shunned this neuroleptic-sparing role, perhaps because of exaggerated fears of tolerance or idiosyncratic disinhibition reactions. A related finding may be the recent report that alprazolam can enhance the antipsychotic effects of antipsychotic compounds, such as fluphenazine, in acutely psychotic patients (Wolkowitz et al., 1988).

# Doses

One fact that has emerged from pharmacokinetic studies of benzodiazepines is that plasma concentrations attained from the same dose vary enormously between individuals. So does their clinical response to such doses. Doses should be carefully titrated by the patient's clinical response. It is usually better to start with the lowest possible dose and increase it as needed rather than start with a dose that may be instantly effective but prove over the long run to be too large. Determining the minimally effective hypnotic dose is a reasonable way to titrate patients' responses. A minimally effective hypnotic dose is one that when taken 2 to 3 hours before bedtime causes the patient to retire earlier, produces a good night of sleep (by whatever criteria the patient uses), and produces only a mild degree of morning sedation. By starting with the lowest possible dose unit and doubling doses each night, one can explore an eightfold range of doses over four nights. In the treatment of anxiety this minimally effective hypnotic dose becomes the major daily dose, with smaller additional doses being given during the day as required. Some representative daily doses of benzodiazepines are shown in Table 2-4.

# Dosage Schedules

Drugs with long elimination half-lives are well-suited to single daily dosage. Such a dosage schedule is desirable for antianxiety drugs, as one does not wish unduly to emphasize drug-taking behavior. The most appropriate time to give single doses is in the evening, when one can also take advantage of the hypnotic effects of these drugs. A patient with anxiety so severe that drug treatment is required commonly has difficulty sleeping. Furthermore, it does not make much pharmacologic sense to instruct patients to take a sedative right after their morning coffee. The "daytime hangover," which is inevitable with the longer-acting drugs, may provide the precise degree of sedation compatible with unimpaired daily activities and relief of troublesome symptoms. Short-acting drugs will require dosing several times a day, and for some patients, the placebo effect of taking medication frequently may be useful.

**Table 2-4. Doses of Some Commonly Used Anxiolytics**

| Drug | Dose mg/day |
|---|---|
| Alprazolam (Xanax) | 0.75–4 |
| Chlordiazepoxide (Librium) | 15–100 |
| Clonazepam (Rivotril) | 1–3 |
| Clorazepate (Tranxene) | 15–60 |
| Diazepam (Valium, Stezolid) | 4–40 |
| Halazepam (Paxipam) | 20–160 |
| Lorazepam (Temesta, Activan) | 2–6 |
| Oxazepam (Serax) | 30–180 |
| Prazepam (Respam, Centrax) | 15–30 |
| Buspirone (Buspar) | 5–40 |

Flexible dosage schedules are generally appreciated by patients. In one study, patients were instructed to ask for counseling and/or diazepam as their symptoms required. The use of drug was reduced over the daily dose that would have ordinarily been prescribed (Winstead et al., 1974). In a survey of chronic users of diazepam (median duration more than 5 years) in which steady-state plasma concentrations of diazepam/nordiazepam were measured, about one-third of patients had concentrations so low as to cast doubt as to their adhering to the prescribed dosage pattern. Many of them were in a range that would be considered subtherapeutic, suggesting that the drug was being taken on an "as needed" basis. None of the patients appeared to be abusing the drug (Hollister et al., 1981).

In the case of buspirone, which requires sustained treatment to attain its subtle effect and which has a short plasma half-life, divided daily doses of at least three to four times a day are necessary. The lack of sedative action permits these divided doses to be equal throughout the day.

## Duration of Treatment

Anxiety is often episodic, waxing and waning with changes in one's life. In such cases, treatment should follow the course of symptoms. Drugs are used only when the patient's symptoms are discomforting or disabling, and never indefinitely. Typical episodes of treatment might be limited to a week or two. If the patient's anxiety is relieved, it probably will remain so in the future without drugs. The knowledge that relief is available when needed may even sustain the patient during subsequent periods of anxiety.

The physician should explain that antianxiety drugs are used for brief, interrupted courses of treatment at the onset of treatment. It is virtually impossible to make this proposal after the patient has been under treatment for several weeks or months and feels fine. Arguments that might be used to persuade patients to follow this course are that tolerance and dependence may develop to the effects of the drug; that is, larger doses will be needed and the patient may be at risk for undergoing withdrawal. Although these arguments apply to only a few patients who take large amounts of drug, most people are so fearful of becoming dependent on drugs that they can be persuasive.

Not all patients who complain of anxiety have the episodic variety. Some patients have chronic symptoms that probably represent an unusually high level of trait anxiety. These patients often do very well with small doses of some antianxiety drug maintained indefinitely. Generally, one need not worry about severe physical dependence developing in such patients, although undoubtedly they may develop some degree of psychological and physical dependence on the drug. Such patients with chronic anxiety are best suited for treatment with buspirone. After taking buspirone, patients have little or no sense of calming or sedation. Some patients actually experience agitation that resembles increased anxiety. The beneficial effects appear gradually and are less noticed by the patient than by those around him. Because of this delay in onset of beneficial effects, patients previously treated with benzodiazepines should be gradually weaned from these drugs over a period of two to three weeks after treatment with buspirone has been initiated. Long-term treatment with buspirone has not yet been associated with any signs of dependence.

The drug label for many benzodiazepines indicates that their efficacy for more than 4 months "has not been assessed by systematic clinical studies." This wording has been widely misinterpreted as indicating that the drugs are not effective for more than 4 months. It means exactly what it says, that such studies simply have not been done. Clinical experience indicates that efficacy may be retained over very long periods.

## Drug Combinations

It makes no sense to combine antianxiety drugs. However, inadvertent combinations can occur when the physician prescribes one drug for use during the day as an anxiolytic, while another is used at night for sleep. As noted earlier, the benzodiazepines are often specifically advertised as anxiolytics or hypnotics, despite their inherent similarity.

Many clinicians now combine beta-adrenoreceptor blocking drugs, such as propranolol, with benzodiazepines. The former drugs allay the somatic aspects of anxiety whereas the latter are more specific for the psychic components. In this sense, the beta blockers may be considered as "benzodiazepine-sparing" agents. Although the practice is widespread, experimental validation of its benefit is lacking.

A combination of chlordiazepoxide and amitriptyline is marketed commercially for the treatment of depression. The addition of the benzodiazepine may hasten the relief of anxiety and insomnia in patients with depression, a favorable property early on in treatment. On the other hand, when full antidepressant doses of amitriptyline are required, the amount of chlordiazepoxide in the combination can become excessive, forcing decreases in the dose to inadequate levels. As with many such combination drugs, the compounds can be given individually just as easily, while allowing the physician to control their ratio.

A case might be made for combining benzodiazepines and buspirone in patients being switched from the former drugs to the latter. A gradual tapering of the benzodiazepine would be expected to avoid withdrawal or rebound symptoms while maintaining some anxiolysis until such time as the therapeutic effect of buspirone may become evident.

## Concomitant Nondrug Treatments

Anxiety is clearly related to life experiences. Thus psychotherapy and altering the environment may be more to the point than drugs in treating anxiety. The word *psychotherapy* is used frequently, but you should be aware that it has almost as many meanings as practitioners. Some purists have maintained that it is impossible to have effective psychotherapy in the presence of drug treatment, as the presence of anxiety is one of the motivating forces for change in psychotherapy. However, little proof exists for this assertion.

Two nonpharmacologic treatments that have much to commend them (they are as effective as any others and have the virtue of being cheap) are exercise and meditation. Exercise can be of any type, from running or walking to swimming or bicycling. Preferably, it should be taken several hours before bedtime. All it costs is calories, something most of us can easily spare. Meditation requires nothing more than a quiet place and some time. No one need pay for a custom-made nonsense syllable as a mantra, as any simple word, such as "one," will do when repeated endlessly.

## Principles of Use

Some general principles of use of antianxiety drugs, based on the foregoing discussion, are listed in Table 2-5.

## NEW PHARMACOLOGIC APPROACHES

Although propranolol was first proposed for treating anxiety in 1966, its use still remains controversial. Literature on the subject has been growing over the years, and results have ranged from ineffective to questionable to effective. Part of this uncertainty is due to the possibility that anxiety may have distinct "psychic" and "somatic" components, with only the latter being affected by the beta-blockers (Ananth and Lin, 1986).

The use of beta-blockers for the treatment of anxiety is consistent with the sympathomimetic model of anxiety discussed previously. Also in line with this model, there has been renewed interest in the use of alpha-2 adrenoreceptor agonists as antianxiety drugs. Such compounds should decrease the firing rate of neurons in the locus coeruleus via presynaptic autoreceptors. Several years ago, a double-blind crossover design in 23 patients treated with clonidine or placebo showed that the drug was effective in those patients who could tolerate it, but that several patients (17 percent) became worse. The main effect of this drug,

**Table 2-5. Summary Principles in Use of Antianxiety Drugs**

1. Use only for good reasons—severe symptoms, disability, discomfort.
2. Be aware that anxiety is only a symptom; try to discern accurate diagnosis before treating.
3. Consider nondrug therapies—psychotherapy, environmental manipulations, exercise, meditation.
4. Propose brief, interrupted courses of treatment at the onset.
5. Titrate doses to the needs of individual patients; avoid oversedation.
6. Constantly assess efficacy—poor efficacy, possibly another diagnosis.
7. Avoid use in those with history of alcohol or drug abuse; buspirone may be drug of choice.
8. Warn patients about interaction with alcohol and other depressants; not necessary with buspirone.
9. Limit number of refills; amounts should be consonant with dosage schedule.
10. Discontinue gradually if the patient has been on therapeutic doses for more than 1 month; not necessary with buspirone.

unlike propranolol, was relief of the psychic but not the somatic symptoms of anxiety (Hoehn-Saric et al., 1981). It should be kept in mind that clonidine is also a weak alpha-1 agonist and that the relative nonspecificity of clonidine may obscure its antianxiety effects. Besides tolerance to its antianxiety action, clonidine may also produce lassitude and hypotension.

If buspirone becomes as much a commercial and clinical success as its sponsors hope, one can be sure that many other modifications of this structure will be studied. Several now only have numbers while others, such as gepirone, have names. Thus far, it appears that these compounds share buspirone's property of being a $5HT_{1A}$ ligand, although they may not have dopaminergic effects similar to buspirone (Peroutka, 1985). The chemical structures of buspirone and related compounds are shown in Figure 2.5.

Other drugs currently under investigation as potential antianxiety compounds include the modified butyrophenone, melperone; several members of the cyclopyrrolone family, which possess a pharmacologic profile similar to benzodiazepines; a mixed benzodiazepine receptor agonist and antagonist; and $5-HT_2$ receptor antagonists, such as ritanserin. Ritanserin, which has already established a reputation as an antihypertensive, seems to produce less side effects than lorazepam (Ceulemans et al., 1985).

# DRUG INTERACTIONS
## Pharmacodynamic

Interactions of antianxiety drugs with other central nervous system depressants are the most important pharmacodynamic interaction. The greatest hazard is that such a combination of drugs will produce oversedation and impaired psychomotor function, respiratory depression, or even unintentional suicide. Impaired function is especially important with regard to driving automobiles—a potentially lethal activity. Interactions with drugs other than those that are sedatives should also be considered. Excessive coffee intake or concurrent use of an appetite suppressant may negate the desired therapeutic effects of the antianxiety drug. Indeed, animal experiments indicate that caffeine may be a direct antagonist of several central effects of diazepam, possibly via a purinergic mechanism (Polc et al., 1981).

## Pharmacokinetic

An interaction with cimetidine has been described for at least two benzodiazepines, and as benzodiazepines and cimetidine both remain among the most widely prescribed drugs in the United States, co-administration of these drugs may well occur. Cimetidine may impair both the dealkylation and oxidation of benzodiazepines by hepatic microsomal enzymes. Delayed clearance of diazepam was found in the presence of cimetidine, and steady-state levels of diazepam were increased by about 40 to 50 percent when cimetidine was added (Klotz and Reimann, 1981). A similar impairment was found with chlordiazepoxide, but not with drugs such as oxazepam and lorazepam, which are only conjugated to glucuronide. If the patient is overly sedated and cannot be switched to one of these latter drugs, a simple way to deal with this situation would be to reduce the dose or increase the dosing interval. Similar pharmacokinetic interactions are possible between benzodiazepines and disulfiram, alcohol, and isoniazid.

# SIDE EFFECTS AND COMPLICATIONS
## Oversedation

Oversedation is the most common side effect of antianxiety drugs. Directing patients to take the largest dose in the evening hours converts this effect from something harmful to something beneficial. Patients should be warned about the possibility of sedation from any dose taken during the day. Usually it will be the greatest 1 to 2 hours after the drug is taken. Activities that would be dangerous, such as driving an automobile or making critical judgments, should be deferred.

## Tolerance/Dependence

Although tolerance readily develops to the sedative effects of benzodiazepines, it may develop slowly or not at all to the antianxiety effects (Rickels et al., 1984). The key to the development of classic tolerance is chronic, uninterrupted use of any drug. The recommendation given before for using these drugs in brief, interrupted courses has the potential for minimizing or avoiding the development of tolerance.

Physical dependence was first described following high multiples of the usual daily dose for both chlordiazepoxide and diazepam, simultaneously with their introduction (Hollister et al., 1961; Hollister et al., 1963).

The major difference with these drugs as compared with the rapid onset of withdrawal from alcohol or short-acting benzodiazepines was the delay in onset, presumably because of their long half-life. Since these early experimental studies in humans, a number of clinical reports of spontaneous dependence on benzodiazepines have appeared, but these are comparatively rare in relationship to the wide use of these drugs. In addition, the majority of these patients became dependent in the context of concurrent abuse of alcohol and other drugs. Cases of genuine physical dependence and withdrawal were much less commonly encountered than cases of presumed psychological dependence (Marks, 1978). The experience of a large mental hospital in Germany indicated that of 33,000 admissions during the period 1974 to 1983, only 150 (0.5 percent) were for benzodiazepine dependence (Laux and Konig, 1987). Presumably, most cases do not merit inpatient treatment.

With the increasing use of shorter-acting benzodiazepines, more severe benzodiazepine withdrawal syndromes are being reported. Seizures and acute delirium have been reported after the abrupt discontinuation of alprazolam. Interestingly, alprazolam withdrawal may be managed by the use of clonidine (Vinogradov et al., 1986) as well as by longer-acting benzodiazepines.

Because the time course of the withdrawal syndrome from drugs such as chlordiazepoxide and diazepam is highly different from that for the shorter-acting barbiturates, such as secobarbital sodium, symptoms and signs often are not evident until the third day following cessation of the drug. They commonly resemble the symptoms initially being treated: nervousness, irritability, and insomnia, so that many patients construe these symptoms as a recrudescence of the anxiety for which they originally took the drug (Power et al., 1985). By either resuming taking their medication, by taking another sedative, or by taking alcohol, they then abort the incipient withdrawal reaction. Others may endure the complete withdrawal reaction without realizing what is wrong. The peak of symptoms from withdrawal of these long-lived drugs occurs at about the fifth day of cessation of the drug; almost all symptoms and signs have disappeared by the eighth or ninth day. Thus, the milder and attenuated withdrawal syndrome from these drugs may be missed, something unlikely to occur with the abrupt and severe withdrawal reaction from short-acting nonbenzodiazepines, such as meprobamate or secobarbital sodium (Ladewig, 1984).

The general rule, then, is that any sedative drug with a plasma disappearance rate of between 6 and 24 hours is most likely to show a severe withdrawal reaction, whereas those with effective disappearance rates (of parent drug as well as active metabolites) of 36 hours or more are likely to have a mild but attenuated withdrawal syndrome. Drugs with a very slow disappearance rate, such as phenobarbital, lack a withdrawal syndrome entirely, as its occurrence is dependent on the rate of declining plasma and tissue drug concentrations.

Although "classic" dependence on benzodiazepines seems to be rare, both in the context of medical as well as nonmedical use, a new phenomenon has been described during the past several years that may be far more common. So-called "therapeutic-dose dependence" on benzodiazepines has been noted with doses within the acceptable therapeutic limits, but that have been continued for months or years. Initial reports of this syndrome were scattered, but the number has greatly increased since an experimental study in 1973 (Covi et al., 1973). Unlike classic dependence, in which doses are fairly large but exposure may be brief, duration of exposure may be the critical variable in therapeutic-dose dependence.

One assumes that the estimate of 1.6 percent of adults in the United States who use benzodiazepines steadily for at least 1 year become dependent is correct. Although the dose × duration parameters of therapeutic-dose dependence are unknown, if we assume that taking benzodiazepines continually for as long as a year might be associated with a high prevalence of such dependence, then the number of persons at risk must be measured in the millions. Those at risk are also those who seem to have the greatest medical need for these agents. However, just because patients receive regular prescriptions of benzodiazepines over long periods of time does not confirm their continual use. About 50 percent of patients considered to be long-term continual users of the drugs actually used them intermittently (Rickels et al., 1984). Whether such intermittent use over long periods of time would mitigate potential withdrawal reactions is unknown. However, the duration of exposure to produce therapeutic-dose dependence may be relatively short. Withdrawal symptoms have appeared following only 6 weeks of exposure to diazepam (Murphy et al., 1984).

It is said that the time-course of withdrawal is likely to be characterized by the early appearance of severe symptoms that then rapidly improve, whereas a recrudescence of symptoms is more likely to be less severe, more gradual in onset, and sustained. Although this time-course difference is definitely the case with classic withdrawal, it has not been so obvious with therapeutic-dose withdrawal. Another confounding variable, at least in humans, is the develop-ment of psychological dependence due to being on a drug that afforded relief of symptoms and then knowing that the same drug has been withdrawn. For instance, patients switched to placebo had less withdrawal symptoms than patients who had all medications suddenly discontinued (Pecknold et al., 1982).

The concept of dependence produced by sedative drugs given at therapeutic doses is still relatively new. The mechanism of action is not clear. One might speculate that in the case of drugs that act on receptors, such as the ben-zodiazepines, prolonged use may cause subsensitivity of receptors. When the drug is withdrawn, the response to any endogenous ligand might be reduced. Furthermore, the possibility exists that patients who require these drugs on a continuing basis are inherently deficient in such endogenous ligands. Such patients might be less protected against sudden withdrawal of their drug, even though it is given to them at modest doses. Of course, all this speculation has no substantial evidence as yet to support it.

## Disinhibition

Outbursts of aggressive or hostile behavior during treatment with various benzodiazepines have been rare, but were described early in their history. In some persons, this undoubtedly represents the release of underlying personality characteristics. Recently, with the rapidly increasing use of alprazolam, several such instances of disinhibition have been reported. However, the behavior observed in some patients has been almost hypomanic in nature (Strahan et al., 1985) (see below).

Depression in patients on these drugs is more than likely coincidental, as nothing in their known pharmacologic actions should be intrinsically depres-sogenic. As discussed earlier, anxiety and depression are frequently inextricable. The depression becomes unmasked as the anxiety is relieved.

## Miscellaneous Adverse Effects

With drugs so widely used as the benzodiazepines are, it would not be surprising if many adverse effects continued to be reported that were not emphasized before. Most of these make pharmacologic sense.

Amnesic effects of these drugs are desired when they are used as anesthetics or adjuncts to anesthesia; in other situations these effects are considered to be adverse. Virtually all benzodiazepines produce amnesia, but whether or not specific members of the class are more likely to do this than others remains unknown. Benzodiazepines cause a dose-related impairment in the acquisition of new information presented during the acute effects. It is not at all certain that such impairment persists with long-term use. They do not affect retention and may facilitate retrieval. Nor do they affect semantic memory or the acquisition of skills. State-dependent learning is a small and inconsequential effect (Lister, 1985).

Several isolated reports of true mania induced by alprazolam make this drug seem different from other benzodiazepines. Perhaps this difference is because other members of the class are seldom used as sole treatments or in large doses for patients with depression. Both tricyclic antidepressant and monoamine oxidase (MAO) inhibitors have been known to exacerbate episodes of mania in depressed patients without previous such episodes. One assumes that these patients have latent bipolar illness. Oddly, the production of mania by alprazolam has been adduced as evidence that it may have a true antidepressant action (Arana et al., 1985).

When high doses of diazepam (100 mg/day) were used in 27 schizophrenic patients previously treated with antipsychotics, 4 developed manifestations of Parkinson syndrome. It has been known for a long while that sedative-hypnotic drugs aggravate Parkinson's disease. One would assume that they might also aggravate a latent drug-induced Parkinson syndrome (Suranyi-Cadotte et al., 1985).

The predisposition to hip fracture in elderly patients taking sedative drugs was confirmed by a large case-control study for benzodiazepines. A significantly increased risk of hip fracture (1.3 to 2.4) was associated with use of sedative–hypnotics with long half-lives (24 hours or more) but not with short half-life drugs. A similar increased risk was found for use of tricyclic antidepressants and antipsychotics. Presumably the sedative effects of these drugs, combined with the autonomic effects of the antidepressants and antipsychotics, make elderly patients more vulnerable to falls (Ray et al., 1987).

Buspirone is notably free of sedative effects. In fact, its side-effects profile includes somewhat opposite effects, such as nervousness and insomnia. Four patients experienced an increase in anxiety levels, agitation, restlessness, pressured speech, and racing thoughts following treatment with buspirone; all had previously been treated with alprazolam (Liegghio et al., 1988). A single patient was treated with three doses of buspirone and within 12 hours of the first dose experienced dramatic myoclonus, dystonias, and akathisia. This sort of reaction is somewhat similar to what one might expect from drugs that are dopamine antagonists (Ritchie et al., 1988).

## Dysmorphogenesis

The issue of dysmorphogenesis is continually raised with all drugs, including the benzodiazepines. It is not yet resolved, as the possible risks are so small as to be unlikely to be detected clinically. Whenever there is doubt, it is wise to be prudent; drugs of any sort should be used only when imperative if the patient is known to be pregnant. If benzodiazepines have been used in a pregnant patient, they should be discontinued if possible as soon as the pregnancy is discovered.

## Overdose

The safety of benzodiazepines in overdose cannot be denied. An extensive survey of 27 medical examiner or coroner offices in the United States and Canada was conducted during the latter part of 1976. The combined jurisdictional population of these sites was 79.2 million people. Diazepam was found to be present on toxicologic analysis in 1239 cases of death. Drugs alone caused death in 914 cases; the remaining 375 fatalities were due to other causes. Only two patients died after having taken only diazepam (Finkle et al., 1980). Considering that one is always at some risk of death whenever one is comatose and treatment is delayed, this minute number of deaths is probably an irreducible minimum for drug overdose.

The use of psychotropic drugs for suicidal purposes may be less frequent than imagined. In a survey done in New Zealand, the rate of such use in patients aged 10 years or older was 3 per 1000 who were prescribed such drugs. Surprisingly, almost three-quarters of those who took overdoses received further prescriptions during the 3 months after their admission to the hospital (Skegg et al., 1983).

## REFERENCES

Alho H, Costa E, Ferrero P, et al (1985) Diazepam-binding inhibitor: a neuropeptide located in selected neural populations of rat brain. Science 229:179–181

Ananth J, Lin KM (1986) Propranolol in psychiatry: therapeutic uses and side effects. Neuropsychobiology 15:20–27

Arana GW, Pearlman C, Shader RI (1985) Alprazolam-induced mania: two clinical cases. Am J Psychiatry 142:368–369

Ballenger JC, Burrows GD, Dupont RL Jr, et al (1988) Alprazolam in panic disorder and agoraphobia: results from a multicenter trial. I. Efficacy in short-term treatment. Arch Gen Psychiatry 45:413–422

Balter MB, Levine J, Manheimer DI (1974) Cross-national study of the extent of antianxiety/sedative drugs use. N Engl J Med 290:769–774

Bellantuono C, Reggi V, Tognoni G, Garattini S (1980) Benzodiazepines: clinical pharmacology and therapeutic use. Drugs 19:195–219

Ceulemans DLS, Hoppenbrouwers ML, Gelders YG, Reyntjens AJM (1985) The influence of ritanserin, a serotonin antagonist, in anxiety disorders: a double-blind placebo-controlled study versus lorazepam. Pharmacopsychiatry 18:293–322

Charney DS, Heninger GR (1986a) Alpha-2-adrenergic and opiate receptor blockade. Arch Gen Psychiatry 43:1037–1041

Charney DS, Heninger GR (1986b) Abnormal regulation of noradrenergic function in panic disorders. Arch Gen Psychiatry 43:1042–1054

Colburn WA, Jack ML (1987) Relationships between CSF drug concentrations, receptor binding characteristics, and pharmacokinetic and pharmacodynamic properties of selected 1,4-substituted benzodiazepines. Clin Pharmacokinet 13:179–190

Costa E (1988) Polytypic signaling at GABAergic synapses. Life Sci 42:1407–1417

Covi L, Lipman RS, Pattison JH, et al (1973) Length of treatment with anxiolytic sedatives and response to their sudden withdrawal. Acta Psychiatr Scand 49:51–64

Ellinwood EH Jr, Heatherly DG, Nikaido AM, et al (1985) Comparative pharmacokinetics and pharmacodynamics of lorazepam, alprazolam and diazepam. Psychopharmacol 86:392–399

Finkle BS, McCloskey KL, Goodman LS (1980) Diazepam and drug associated deaths in a United States and Canada survey. JAMA 242:429–434

Garakani H, Zitrin CM, Klein DF (1984) Treatment of panic disorder with imipramine alone. Am J Psychiatry 141:446–448

Greenblatt DJ, Shader RI (1985) Clinical pharmacokinetics of the benzodiazepines. p. 43–58 In Smith DE, Wesson DR, (eds): The Benzodiazepines: Current Standards for Medical Practice. MTP Press, Lancaster, UK

Guentert TW (1984) Time-dependence in benzodiazepine pharmacokinetics. Mechanisms and clinical significance. Clin Pharmacokinet 9:203–210

Haefely W (1985) Biochemistry of anxiety. Ann Acad Med (Singapore) 14:81–83

Henauer SA, Gallaher EJ, Hollister LE (1984) Long-lasting single-dose tolerance to neurologic deficits induced by diazepam. Psychopharmacol 82:161–163

Hoehn-Saric R, Merchant AF, Keyser ML, Smith VK (1981) Effects of clonidine on anxiety disorders. Arch Gen Psychiatry 38:1278–1282

Hollister LE (1984) Selection of benzodiazepines. JDR J Drug Ther Res 9:416–422

Hollister LE, Bennett JL, Kimbell I Jr, et al (1963) Diazepam in newly admitted schizophrenics. Dis Nervous System 24:1–4

Hollister LE, Conley FK, Britt RH, Shuer L (1981) Long-term use of diazepam. JAMA 246:1568–1570

Hollister LE, Motzenbecker FP, Degan RO (1961) Withdrawal reactions from chlordiazepoxide ("Librium"). Psychopharmacol 2:63–68

Klotz U, Reimann I (1981) Elevation of steady-state diazepam levels by cimetidine. Clin Pharmacol Ther 30:513–517

Lader M (1987) Assessing the potential for buspirone dependence and abuse and effects of withdrawal. Am J Med 82 (suppl 5A):20–26

Ladewig D (1984) Dependence liability of the benzodiazepines. Drug Alcohol Depend 13:139–149

Laux G, Konig W (1987) Long-term use of benzodiazepines in psychiatric patients. Acta Psychiatr Scand 76:64–70

Liegghio NE, Yergani UK, Moore NC (1988) Buspirone-induced jitteriness in three patients with panic disorder and one patient with generalized anxiety disorder. J Clin Psychiatry 44;165–166

Lister RG (1985) The amnesic action of benzodiazepines in man. Neurosci Biobehavioral Rev 9:87–94

Marks J (1978) The Benzodiazepines: Use, Misuse, Abuse. MPT Press, Lancaster, UK, p 111

Martin IL (1987) The benzodiazepines and their receptors: 25 years of progress. Neuropharmacol 26:957–970

Mason ST, Fibiger HC (1979) I. Anxiety: the locus coeruleus disconnection. Life Sci 25:2141–2147

Mellinger GD, Balter MB, Manheimer DI, et al (1978) Psychic distress, life crisis, and use of psychotherapeutic medications. National household survey. Arch Gen Psychiatry 35:1045–1052

Mellinger GD, Balter MB, Uhlenhuth EH (1984) Prevalence and correlates of the longterm regular use of anxiolytics. Arch Gen Psychiatry 251:375–379

Mohler H, Okada T (1977) Benzodiazepine receptor: demonstration in the central nervous system. Science 198:859–861

Mohler H, Richards JG (1981) Agonist and antagonist benzodiazepine receptor interaction in vitro. Nature (London) 294:763–765

Murphy SM, Owen RT, Tyrer PJ (1984) Withdrawal symptoms after six weeks' treatment with diazepam. Lancet 2:1389

Myers JK, Weissman MM, Tischler GL, et al (1984) Six-month prevalence of psychiatric disorders in three communities. 1980 to 1983. Arch Gen Psychiatry 41:959–967

Noyes R, Anderson DJ, Clancey J, et al (1984) Diazepam and propranolol in panic disorder and agoraphobia. Arch Gen Psychiatry 41:287–292

Olajida D, Lader M (1987) A comparison of buspirone, diazepam, and placebo in patients with chronic anxiety states. J Clin Psychopharmacol 7:148–152

Palmer DP (1988) Buspirone, a new approach to the treatment of anxiety. FASEB J 2:2445–2452

Pecknold JC, Familamiri P, Chang H, et al (1985) Buspirone: anxiolytic? Prog Neuropsychopharmacol Biol Psychiatry 9:639–642

Pecknold JC, McClure DJ, Fleuri D, Chang H (1982) Benzodiazepine withdrawal effects. Prog Neuropsychopharmacol Biol Psychiatry 6:517–722

Peroutka SJ (1985) Selective interaction of novel anxiolytics with 5-hydroxytryptamine 1A receptors. Biol Psychiatry 20:971–979

Polc P, Bonetti EP, Pieri L, et al (1981) Caffeine antagonizes several central effects of diazepam. Life Sci 28:2265–2275

Power KG, Jerrom DWA, Simpson RJ, Mitchell M (1985) Controlled study of withdrawal symptoms and rebound anxiety after six week course of diazepam for generalized anxiety. Br Med J 290:1246–1248

Rapoport JL (1988) The neurobiology of obsessive-compulsive disorder. JAMA 260:2888–2890

Ray WA, Griffin MR, Schaffner W, et al (1987) Psychotropic drug use and the risk of hip fracture. N Engl J Med 316:363–369

Rickels K, Case GW, Winokur A, Swenson C (1984) Longterm benzodiazepine therapy: risks and benefits. Psychopharmacol Bull 20:608–615

Ritchie EC, Bridenbaugh RH, Jabbari B (1988) Acute generalized myoclonus following buspirone administration. J Clin Psychiatry 47:242–243

Robins LN, Helzer JE, Weissman MM, et al (1984) Lifetime prevalence of specific psychiatric disorders in three sites. Arch Gen Psychiatry 41:949–958

Saletu B, Pakesch G (1987) Recent advances in the clinical pharmacology of benzodiazepines. Part I: Pharmacokinetics. Hum Psychopharmacol 2:3–10

Sanghera MK, McMillen BA, German DC (1983) Buspirone, a non-benzodiazepine anxiolytic, increases locus coeruleus noradrenergic neuronal activity. Eur J Pharmacol 86:107–110

Sheehan DV, Ballenger J, Jacobsen C (1980) Treatment of endogenous anxiety with phobic, hysterical, and hypochondriacal symptoms. Arch Gen Psychiatry 37:51–59

Skegg K, Skegg DCG, Richards SM (1983) Incidence of self-poisoning in patients prescribed psychotropic drugs. Br Med J 286:841–843

Skolnick P, Moncada V (1981) Pentobarbital: dual actions to increase brain benzodiazepine receptor affinity. Science 211:1448–1450

Squires RF, Braestrup C (1977) Benzodiazepine receptors in rat brain. Nature 266:732–734

Strahan A, Rosenthal J, Kaswan M, Winston A (1985) Three case reports of acute paroxysmal excitement associated with alprazolam treatment. Am J Psychiatry 142:859–861

Suranyi-Cadotte BE, Nestoros JN, Nair PV, et al (1985) Parkinsonism induced by high doses of diazepam. Biol Psychiatry 20:451–460

Tallman Jr, Paul SM, Skolnick P, Gallagher DW (1980) Receptors for the age of anxiety: pharmacology of the benzodiazepines. Science 207:274–281

Taylor DP (1988) Buspirone, a new approach to the treatment of anxiety. FASEB J 2:2445–2452

Thompson WL, Johnson AD, Maddrey WL, Osler Housestaff (1975) Diazepam and paraldehyde for treatment of severe delirium tremens. Ann Intern Med 82:175–180

Tyrer P, Treasaden I, Moreton K, et al (1984) Value of serum diazepam and nordiazepine measurements in anxious patients. J Affective Disord 7:1–10

Vinogradov S, Reiss AL, Csernansky JC (1986) Clonidine therapy in withdrawal from high-dose alprazolam treatment. Am J Psychiatry 143:1188

Wilensky AJ, Ojemann LM, Temkin NR, et al (1981) Clorazepate and phenobarbital as antiepileptic drugs: a double-blind study. Neurology (NY) 31:1271–1276

Williams VC, Varnado GC, Nwangwu PU (1985) Perspectives on the clinical pharmacology of benzodiazepines. Drugs Today 21:75–96

Wilson J, Ellis FR (1973) Oral premedication with lorazepam (Ativan): a comparison with heptabarbitone (Medomin) and diazepam (Valium). Br J Anaesth 45:738–744

Winstead DK, Anderson A, Eilers MK, et al (1974) Diazepam on demand: drug-seeking behavior in psychiatric inpatients. Arch Gen Psychiatry 30:349–351

Wolkowitz OM, Breier A, Doran A, et al (1988) Alprazolam augmentation of antipsychotic effect of fluphenazine in schizophrenic patients. Arch Gen Psychiatry 45:664–672

# 3

---

# HYPNOTICS

## HISTORY

Hypnotics are drugs that promote sleep and inhibit wakefulness. Seldom do usual doses enforce sleep, that is, make rested subjects not prepared to sleep fall asleep against their will. Thus, these drugs are used merely as adjuncts to facilitate a normal process. Sleep deprivation remains the most powerful influence for inducing sleep.

Historically, many different drugs have been used. The name of morphine originated from its apparent ability to cause sleep, although it has seldom been used for this purpose. Paraldehyde, chloral hydrate, and glutethimide are examples of drugs that have been used as hypnotics in the recent past but that are now considered to be obsolete.

Barbiturates were introduced as hypnotics early in the twentieth century and have been a most enduring group of drugs. Many modifications of their chemical structures have imparted a variety of pharmacologic actions to these drugs. They were certainly the wonder drugs of the psychopharmacology of their time. Many are still used as hypnotics, but use has markedly diminished.

The introduction of the benzodiazepines in 1960 was as revolutionary as the introduction of barbiturates. As they perform many of the same clinical functions and are far safer, many consider other hypnotics to be obsolete. The number of benzodiazepines available for use as hypnotics has increased during the past several years, as has their percentage of the market for hypnotics.

## THE BIOLOGY OF SLEEP

The functions of sleep are unknown. Considering its ubiquity, its complexity, and its peremptory demand, the failure to demonstrate a vital function for sleep is amazing; especially as it may be construed as "wasted time." Sleep may have originated as an instinctual process for conserving energy and affording security (Meddis, 1977). The consequences of sleep loss are known to everyone. Daytime drowsiness, a lack of motivation, and a feeling of dysphoria are common experiences after one or two nights of poor sleep. In animals, sleep deprivation for only a few weeks has been shown to be fatal, suggesting a potentially vital function of sleep (Chase, 1986). However, sleep deprivation studies in humans have failed to produce evidence of a vital need for sleep.

The need for sleep as applied to daily living is most evident by the lack of alertness and the daytime dysphoria that follows a poor night's sleep. However, the amount of sleep required to avoid these consequences is highly individual. The true test of whether someone has attained a satisfactory amount of sleep is how quickly they fall asleep during the day when given an opportunity.

Until fairly recently, sleep was thought to be homogeneous. The fundamental discovery that sleep has variable stages, in which rapid eye movement (REM) sleep is associated with dreaming, was made slightly more than three decades ago. Non-REM sleep, which occupies much more of total sleep time, has been divided into four stages based on electrophysiologic patterns.

Although it is now possible to determine the architecture of sleep in normal or insomniac patients in the sleep laboratory, the meaning of departures from normal patterns, either spontaneous or drug induced, is far from clear. After an initial period of lying awake (sleep latency), normal sleep in a young person begins with stage 1 NREM and then progresses to stage 4 NREM. Once a person has attained stage 4 NREM sleep, this state is periodically interrupted by REM sleep throughout the night. The first episode of REM sleep can be expected to occur within 60 to 90 minutes of the time the individual falls asleep. Further episodes repeat approximately every 90 minutes, and the length of these REM episodes gradually increases. REM sleep somewhat resembles the awake state electrographically; the EEG tracing shows a similar low-voltage, fast activity, but eye movements are more frequent and more regular than in the awake state. The major difference in the REM state is a completely flat electromyogram (EMG) tracing, which indicates marked neuromuscular inhibition, in effect, paralysis.

Brief awakenings may occur from REM or stage 2 NREM sleep. In the elderly, sleep latency is increased and stage 4 NREM sleep may be entirely absent. The onset of the first REM period (REM latency) is also delayed, although REM periods tend to have the same length, and awakenings are more frequent. By continual recording throughout the night, it is possible to distinguish among these various types of sleep, to record the pattern of their occurrence, and to calculate the total amount of time spent in each state (Kales et al., 1969). A "normal" night's sleep is a highly personal phenomenon, which undergoes progressive changes during one's life span.

Extreme swings in many physiologic systems and functions accompany the various sleep stages. During NREM sleep, heart rate and respirations are slowed, blood pressure falls, and body temperature and metabolic activity are decreased. Recently, relationships between body temperature prior to falling asleep and the subsequent amount and quality of NREM sleep, in particular stage 4 NREM sleep, have been of interest. Modest increases in body temperature before sleep, termed thermal loads, increase the amount of stage 4 NREM sleep, whereas larger thermal loads decrease stage 4 NREM sleep (Parmeggiani, 1987). Curiously, this mechanism may explain why ancient remedies for insomnia such as moderate exercise or a warm bedtime bath (Horne and Shackell, 1987) are so successful. During REM sleep, heart and respiratory rate become variable and accelerated; oxygen saturation of blood decreases, along with an increase in oxygen utilization; and penile erection is typical.

Our understanding of sleep must be integrated into an increasingly complex system of circadian rhythms. All circadian biologic rhythms may be driven by one of two main "pacemakers," so-called soft and hard. The soft pacemaker regulates rest–activity rhythms, whereas the hard pacemaker is linked to body temperature rhythms (Moore-Ede et al., 1983). Environmental cues usually entrain these pacemakers to function in concert. However, in the absence of such entrainment, their independent functioning can be observed. Curiously, all aspects of sleep may not be driven by the same pacemaker. Stage 4 NREM sleep occurrence has been linked to the hard pacemaker, whereas the propensity for REM sleep has been linked to the soft pacemaker. The daily alternation of wakefulness and sleep will be viewed one day in the context of an overarching array of biologic rhythms.

The roles of various neurotransmitters in sleep physiology is still being explored. Destruction of the median raphe system and its serotonin-containing neurons markedly diminishes all stages of sleep (Jouvet, 1969). Recently, the length of various sleep stages has been correlated with cerebrospinal fluid concentrations of serotonin's principal metabolite, 5-hydroxyindole acetic acid. When the synthesis of serotonin is blocked by the tryptophan hydroxylase inhibitor, parachlorphenylalanine, insomnia and loss of REM sleep ensue. Administration of 5-hydroxytryptophan, a precursor of serotonin, counters this effect. Increasing brain concentrations of acetylcholine by cholinesterase inhibition with drugs such as physostigmine or arecoline increases REM sleep. Atropine blocks the transition from NREM to REM sleep, suggesting that a cholinergic mechanism may trigger the noradrenergic system of the locus ceruleus. The role of dopamine is still uncertain.

Peptides that promote sleep have been isolated from mammalian brain, as well as from urine and cerebrospinal fluid. These substances have been referred to as substance S. Because these peptides contain residues of muramic acid, an amino acid that forms the backbone of bacterial cell walls, they are called muramyl peptides (Krueger et al., 1986). The concentration of these peptides increases as a consequence of sleep deprivation. They have their greatest effects on the quantity of stage 4 NREM sleep; some of their actions may be mediated by other CNS peptides, such as interleukin 1.

## SLEEP DISORDERS

The classification of sleep disorders is constantly changing. The most recent, in DSM IIIR, recognizes two broad categories, dyssomnias and parasomnias. The former includes insomnia, hypersomnia, and disorders of the sleep–wake cycle.

The latter include aberrations, such as nightmares, sleep terror, and sleep-walking. Other classifications have also been proposed, and it is likely that any offered will be subject to future change.

Insomnia is by far the most common sleep disorder. Hypersomnia tends to be less common and the parasomnias least. The prevalence of disorders of sleep was assessed in a 1979 survey. During the course of a year, 35 percent of adults complained of having insomnia; one-half of these considered the problem to be serious. Older patients and women were more likely to complain of serious insomnia; they also had higher levels of psychic distress, somatic anxiety, symptoms resembling major depression, and multiple health problems. Only 2.6 percent of adults used a medically prescribed hypnotic, but if antianxiety drugs and antidepressants are counted, 4.3 percent used prescribed sleep aids. Another 3.1 percent used an over-the-counter sleeping remedy. The majority of serious insomniacs (85 percent) were untreated by any type of medication (Mellinger et al., 1985).

Insomnia is a complaint about inadequate sleep. The actual amount of sleep may be decreased, or the person may awaken with a sense of being unrested despite an apparently normal amount of sleep. Many people who complain of insomnia are found, after study in the sleep laboratory, to have no sleep disturbance, whereas others may show sleep disorders without a complaint. Nearly everyone has had a few nights of inadequate sleep in their life. This experience is hardly abnormal and requires no specific treatment. The clinical diagnosis of insomnia should only be applied when inadequate sleep occurs several times a week for at least 1 month. When the complaint has existed for 3 months or more, insomnia is said to be chronic.

The diagnosis of sleep disorders relies heavily on the history, including medical, psychiatric, and drug elements. History should also be obtained from a bed partner. Physical examination will only provide confirmation of disorders that may be painful during the night, such as rheumatoid arthritis or peptic ulcer. Ordinary laboratory workup is usually noncontributory. A sleep laboratory workup needs to be done only rarely, as the cost of a single night of study may be as high as $1000.

Some forms of insomnia may be caused by relatively minor disruptions in a person's environment or habits. Persons who travel through several time zones a day may find that their normal biologic rhythms, including that of sleep-awakening, are interrupted. Sleeping in a strange bed or in unusual surroundings may interfere with normal sleep. Any change in the accustomed ambient noise level during the night may temporarily alter one's sleep pattern. Some persons develop poor sleep hygiene, that is, a habitual indulgence in snacks or late night movies in bed may interfere with falling asleep. Finally, some people seem to require less sleep or require it in a more erratic pattern, such as by frequent naps rather than by sustained sleep.

As much as 35 percent of insomnia is thought to be caused by other psychiatric disorders. Simple worry or excitement can interfere with sleep. Such causes are easily uncovered. Chronic anxiety disorders are almost always accompanied by some degree of sleep disturbance, as is depression. Patients who experience insomnia and also complain of diminished interest and energy, loss of weight, weeping, and anxiety need further psychiatric assessment and may eventually respond to treatment for depression. Other complaints of insomniacs should alert the physician to look for physical disorders.

The use of drugs, whether over-the-counter or prescription, are common causes of dyssomnias, and a careful drug history is imperative when evaluating these disorders. Two commonly taken social drugs may interfere with sleep. Caffeine is generally recognized as having this effect, but it may not do so until the middle years of life. Therefore, persons who were always able to drink their evening cup of coffee without suffering sleep problems may begin to find sleep more difficult and fail to associate the insomnia with its ingestion. Although alcohol is a depressant and often enhances the onset of sleep, some degree of sleep disorganization later on in the night is inevitable. Heavy drinkers often find that they awaken in the early morning in a stimulated state. Appetite suppressants of the sympathomimetic type can also interfere with sleep.

Insomnia secondary to hypnotic dependence has been elucidated during the past several years by sleep laboratory studies. Prolonged use of hypnotic drugs results in severe deprivation of REM sleep with marked rebound when attempts are made to discontinue treatment. Sleep may then be of poor quality and punctuated by nightmares and frequent awakening. Thus, treating insomnia inappropriately may produce a new type of disorder. As hypnotics may aggravate the symptoms they treat, those who prescribe them should realize that these drugs could have this potential and should make patients aware of the hazard.

An increasingly frequent cause of insomnia is sleep apnea. It is a universal occurrence in infants and may be related to some cases of sudden infant death syndrome. In adults, its prevalence increases dramatically with age. In addition, being overweight is a risk factor. During periods of sleep apnea, respiration ceases totally. This is due to either a central mechanism from diminished sensitivity of the respiratory center, a peripheral mechanism of upper airway obstruction, or both. When upper airway obstruction occurs, the patient may resume breathing with marked snorting or gasping sounds, so that the diagnosis may be suggested clinically if such sounds were heard by another who shared the same room or bed with the patient. These episodes, which may number in the 100s, cause frequent awakenings that result in poor sleep. The patient's complaint is often one of daytime hypersomnia (Guilleminault et al., 1973). Use of hypnotics, which might further depress respiratory drive, would be clearly contraindicated in such cases of sleep apnea.

Periodic movements in sleep (PMS), formerly called nocturnal myoclonus, is an abnormality in which the patient has myoclonic movements, especially of the lower extremities, throughout the night. They may be relatively mild twitching movements of the anterior tibial area, which disturb sleep without causing full awakening. At the other extreme, they may be kicking movements that may bruise a bed partner and lead to awakening. In the latter instance, the diagnosis can be made by the testimony of the bed partner. Milder instances may only be proved by sleep laboratory studies.

Sleepwalking, sleep terrors, as well as enuresis occur during stage 4 NREM sleep (slow-wave sleep). Enuresis responds well to tricyclic antidepressants, but other procedures should be tried first. Drugs that reduce or eliminate stage 4 NREM sleep, such as benzodiazepines, might be worth trying for sleepwalking or sleep terrors. Sleep terrors are manifested by terrible fragmented nightmare-like experiences, although most anxiety-provoking dreams that lead to voluntary awakenings tend to occur during REM sleep (Hauri, 1975).

# TYPES OF HYPNOTICS

Although specific agents have been selectively promoted as hypnotics, this group of drugs is not particularly distinctive. Most drugs used for treating anxiety (see Chapter 2) could be used equally well as hypnotics. Usually the hypnotic dose of the drug is somewhat higher than the anxiolytic dose, but these actions are similar in nature. Thus, many classifications refer to these drugs as sedative–hypnotic.

## Chemical Structures

For practical purposes, virtually all older hypnotics should be considered as obsolete. The older arguments based on price no longer hold because both flurazepam and temazepam have become generic. Other generic benzodiazepines that could also be used as hypnotics include diazepam, chlordiazepoxide, and lorazepam. If the prudent prescribing practices recommended below are followed, cost should not be an important consideration.

The benzodiazepines are now the most popular hypnotics, and their predominance continues to grow. Flurazepam has had the longest history of use, but newer, short-acting benzodiazepines, such as temazepam and triazolam, have overtaken this older drug in popularity. The structural similarity among these benzodiazepines is evident in Figure 3-1.

Increasing use of benzodiazepines has had the desirable effect of reducing the number of successful suicides from sedative–hypnotic overdose. Benzodiazepines are extraordinarily safe in overdose, and their use as the agent for a suicide attempt is much less likely to be successful. Sadly, the number of drug-induced suicides as a whole has not declined, as those intent on self-destruction find other drugs that will produce the desired result.

## Pharmacologic Properties

Not very much can be said with certainty about the mode or locus of action of benzodiazepines when they are used as hypnotics. A wide variety of brain structures may be involved. The reticular activating system is an obvious locus of action, but the median raphe may also be involved as well as many polysynaptic pathways from the brain stem to the cerebral cortex.

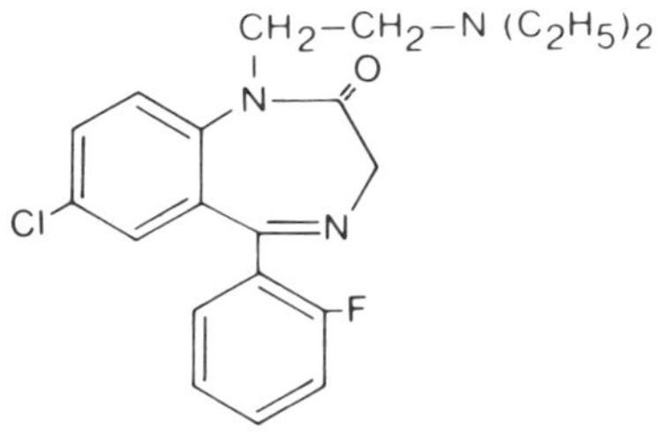

Flurazepam

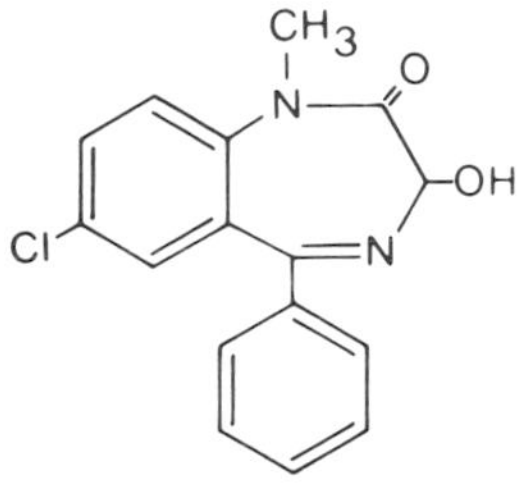

Temazepam

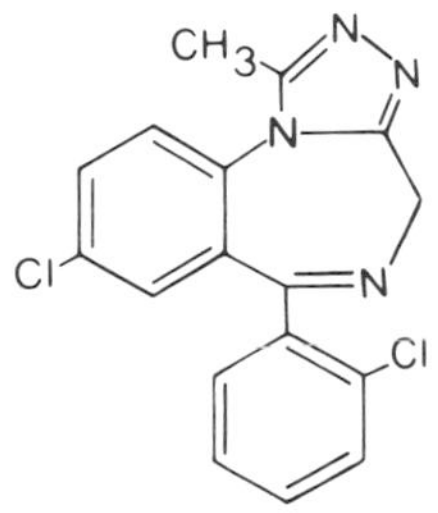

Triazolam

**Fig. 3-1.** Structural relationships between various benzodiazepine hypnotics.

The discovery of benzodiazepine receptors that are linked to GABA receptors and membrane chloride channels may apply to at least one mode of action (see Chapter 2). As GABA is a major CNS inhibitory neurotransmitter, and far more abundant than aminergic neurotransmitters such as serotonin, norepinephrine, and dopamine, it is tempting to explain the action of these drugs in producing gradations of CNS depression (anxiolysis, sedation, hypnosis, anesthesia, coma) to widespread neuronal hyperpolarization (Chweh et al., 1984). However, it seems unlikely that this mechanism will explain the action of all other types of hypnotic drugs, or even totally explain the action of benzodiazepines.

Besides GABA, serotonin may also be important in hypnotic action. Parachlorophenylalanine, which blocks serotonin synthesis, produces insomnia, while presumed serotonin precursors, such as 5-hydroxytryptophan and 1-tryptophan, produce sleep. Serotonin homologs, such as melatonin, can also promote sleep. The role of other aminergic neurotransmitters is far less evident.

As almost all drugs that are classified as sedative–hypnotics have dose-dependent gradations of CNS depression, it is sometimes difficult to explain why some are specifically designated as antianxiety drugs while others are characterized as hypnotics. Most of the time the characterization of a drug as a hypnotic is based either on traditional use or on the indication selected by the pharmaceutical company seeking a market for the drug.

# Pharmacokinetics

In general, drugs that are active in the CNS must have a relatively high lipid-to-water partition coefficient and a low degree of ionization at the body pH. Most hypnotic drugs are weak acids or weak bases that are highly un-ionized at pH 7.4. This favors their passage across the blood-brain barrier.

Because water solubility hastens absorption, most drugs are available as water-soluble salts. Weakly basic drugs, such as the benzodiazepines, are most effectively absorbed at the nearly neutral pH of the small intestine. In any case, absorption is both rapid and nearly complete.

Many hypnotic drugs are bound to plasma proteins, but they are easily distributed to the brain and body tissues. Because these drugs often have low rates of metabolism and minimal renal excretion, the processes by which they are distributed may be more instrumental in terminating their effects than the manner in which they are metabolized. They are metabolized in the liver; usually they are conjugated with a polar group (glucuronide). These drugs are rarely excreted unchanged. The pharmacokinetic properties of three widely used benzodiazepine hypnotics are summarized in Table 3-1. (Greenblatt et al., 1983).

Flurazepam is most different from the other drugs. Virtually none of the parent compound can be detected following oral doses. Two active metabolites are formed, but one, desalkylflurazepam, accounts for virtually all effects (Miller et al., 1988). Although this metabolite appears quickly following oral doses, it has a very long plasma elimination half-life. This long half-life has raised several concerns. First, the drug may have significant sedative carryover effects the next day. Such does not seem to be uniformly the case, however. When next-day sedative side effects of flurazepam were compared with those following the short half-life drug triazolam, they were comparable. As is often the case with long half-life drugs, the prevailing plasma concentrations during the elimination half-life may be so low as to produce little pharmacologic effect. Second, the drug may accumulate with long-term daily use. This danger is real; assuming a mean plasma half-life of 72 hours, steady-state plasma concentrations might not be attained for 12 to 15 days and could be high enough to produce demonstrable effects.

Temazepam is completely absorbed, with peak concentrations following oral doses within 2 to 3 hours. The plasma half-life characterizes it as a short-acting benzodiazepine (Jochemsen et al., 1983). It produces no active metabolites.

### Table 3-1. Pharmacokinetic Parameters of Three Benzodiazepine Hypnotics

| | Cmax (h) | Protein Binding | Active Metabolite | Half-life (h) |
|---|---|---|---|---|
| Flurazepam[a] | 1–3 | 96 | Desalkyl | 40–114 |
| Temazepam | 2–3 | 96 | None | 9.5–12.4 |
| Triazolam | 0.7–2 | 80 | None | 1.3–3.9 |

[a] Data pertain to desalkylflurazepam.

With no active metabolites and a relatively short plasma half-life, cumulation is not a problem. One would think that daytime sedation should not be much of a problem either, but the "hangover" effects of hypnotics are more dependent on the dose given than on the plasma elimination half-life.

Triazolam has virtually no active metabolites and a very short plasma half-life. Thus, it represents the extreme departure from flurazepam, with temazepam occupying the middle ground.

## EFFECT OF HYPNOTICS ON SLEEP LABORATORY MEASUREMENTS

Although the significance of drug-induced deviations from normal sleep electrophysiology patterns is still unclear, one might suppose that the less the departure, the better. No drug has been found yet that does not cause some departure from normal sleep patterns.

Initial hopes that benzodiazepines would have less disruptive effects than the barbiturates on the architecture of sleep have not been realized. Both types of drugs reduce REM and stage 4 sleep. Flurazepam suppresses REM sleep immediately, but this effect dissipates quickly after drug withdrawal; stage 4 NREM suppression is delayed and persists during a 3-day withdrawal period. The actual number of slow waves is not decreased, only the number of epochs that would conventionally be interpreted as slow wave sleep. Thus, the puzzle of why so little clinical effect ensues from a reduction in this presumably critical stage of sleep may be solved (Feinberg et al., 1979).

Criteria for referring patients for sleep laboratory evaluations are still poorly defined. Some would order such a study in any patient who has not responded to treatment and whose insomnia remains essentially undiagnosed and persistent for 4 weeks. On the other hand, there are specific symptoms that should warrant referral. Abnormal respirations and heavy snoring or snorting sounds during the night may indicate sleep apnea, which can be definitely diagnosed in the sleep laboratory. Abnormal movements during sleep, especially of the legs, may indicate PMS, also easily diagnosed in the sleep laboratory. Sleep apnea is a positive contraindication to use of hypnotics whereas PMS can be effectively treated with clonazepam. The extent of what sleep laboratory measurements are made will depend on the particular case.

## CLINICAL USE OF HYPNOTICS
### Desiderata of an Ideal Hypnotic

An ideal hypnotic would produce sleep quickly. Most benzodiazepines are highly lipid-soluble and readily absorbed. However, absorption may be much retarded if the drug is taken and a recumbent position is assumed. An ideal hypnotic should have no hangover effects the next day. Such residual effects are most often due to having taken a dose larger than required. Differences in hangover attributable to differences in plasma half-life are relatively minor. If hangover occurs with benzodiazepines, it can be quickly countered by the caffeine in one's morning cup of coffee. Ideally, hypnotics should have no amnestic activity. This property is inherent with all benzodiazepines. Whether it is greater with triazolam is uncertain, but it is definitely related to dose (Shader and Greenblatt, 1983). One would hope that an ideal hypnotic would not have an additive effect with alcohol. As both benzodiazepines and alcohol are sedatives, this interaction is unavoidable. It is of clinical consequence only when benzodiazepines are taken in suicidal doses, however. One would also like an ideal hypnotic not to produce dependence or have the liability for abuse. Benzodiazepines can do both. Most documentation of dependence has been in patients who take these drugs as anxiolytics several times a day for long periods of time. Reports of dependence following use as hypnotics are far less common.

Although benzodiazepines do not yet meet the desiderata of ideal hypnotics, they do come reasonably close. With prudent use, many of the deficiencies of these drugs can be mitigated. Their current popularity for use as hypnotics is well deserved.

## Importance of Diagnostic Inquiry

Insomnia is a condition of heterogeneous origin. A working diagnosis should always be made before hypnotic drugs are prescribed. The importance of the history cannot be overemphasized. Some diagnoses are readily evident, as when the patient has changed his job and works a different shift. Others may require a bit more probing, as in the depressed patient with a sleep disorder. Still others may be actively concealed by the patient, as in the alcoholic who denies the extent of his or her drinking. One must be certain to rule out the absolute contraindications to the use of hypnotics, which include sleep disturbance associated with chronic obstructive pulmonary disease, drug and alcohol misuse, depression with a high risk of suicide, and pregnancy, as well as sleep apnea.

## Indications

Currently, insomnia may be thought of as having three phases: transient insomnia, short-term insomnia, and long-term insomnia. The amount of diagnostic inquiry required and the readiness with which one prescribes hypnotics will vary with the phase (NIH Consensus Conference, 1984).

Transient insomnia is the primary indication for hypnotics. This state may be induced by a change in surroundings, temporary emotional crisis, jet lag associated with a shift in time zones, or a change in work schedules. Curiously, evaluations of hypnotics are more often accomplished in patients with chronic insomnia, which may lead to the belief that doses and duration of treatment must be great even when hypnotics are used for transient insomnia. In any case, the need for hypnotics will be brief as adjustments are made.

Short-term insomnia usually lasts for less than a month. It may be associated with bereavement or a family crisis, or with some intercurrent medical problem. Use of hypnotics briefly to tide the patient over the temporary sleep disturbance is relatively noncontroversial.

Long-term insomnia is generally defined as insomnia that has lasted 3 months or more. Here one is obliged to do an extensive diagnostic workup. Many cases of long-term insomnia are associated with psychiatric conditions, with drug or alcohol abuse, or with chronic medical problems. To the extent that these contribute to insomnia, their management should take priority over the use of hypnotics. In older patients, sleep apnea or periodic movements may contribute to the problem. If these diagnoses are not strongly suggested clinically (often a bed partner can provide adequate information), sleep laboratory studies might be in order. Nonetheless, even extensive investigation may not discover a suitable explanation for the continuing complaint of insomnia. Hypnotic drugs may afford the best relief but should be used with constraints noted below.

## Treatment of Underlying Disorders

Some patients with insomnia require specific treatment for an underlying disorder. Antidepressants or electroconvulsive therapy may be required in the depressed patient who has insomnia. Schizophrenics are often troubled by insomnia, although it is seldom the presenting complaint. Antipsychotics are often not adequate, in which case hypnotics may be added. Poor sleep due to anxiety should be treated with the same drug used for treating the latter symptom. One need not use two sedative-hypnotics concurrently, such as diazepam in the day and flurazepam at night.

Withdrawal of alcohol or sedative–hypnotics in heavy users may be adequate to relieve insomnia. Antacids or cimetidine may be needed to relieve sleep-disturbing night pain of peptic ulcer. The phase-delay syndrome, in which the patient's biologic rhythms are out of phase with his daily schedule, can be treated by adjusting that schedule.

## Nonpharmacologic Therapy for Insomnia

The relaxation that follows a warm bath, a massage, or the relief of sexual tension can promote sleep. Many insomniacs have developed elaborate rituals for courting sleep, and some seem to work. Boring tasks that do not require close attention, such as watching the many commercials during the late movie on television, can also induce sleep. In fact, it may be worthwhile to plan rituals for patients who seek relief from insomnia and link them with drug therapy in order to take advantage of the conditioned aspect of the process of going to sleep.

A regular pattern of daytime activities and exercise will facilitate normal sleep. Increasing an insomniac's activity level to the point of moderate fatigue may induce sleep. Some patients may merely need to shift their bedtime. A patient who awakens early in the morning after 6 or more hours of sleep should consider retiring later. The distress that ensues when one awakens at 3 or 4 A.M.

and cannot get back to sleep can undo the restorative value of sleep already obtained.

Difficult therapeutic decisions must be made in the patient who has used hypnotics chronically without evidence of abuse. Chronic use may be avoided by encouraging the concurrent use of nondrug approaches to treatment. If such patients have not been previously treated with nonpharmacologic methods, they should be tried. Patients who relapse following discontinuation of hypnotics and who once again benefit when they are restarted may deserve continued treatment, even though it is not the ideal.

## Choice of Drug

Benzodiazepines are now the preferred hypnotic drugs. The continued use of drugs such as the barbiturates glutethimide, methprylon, ethchlorvynol, and others cannot be justified, as each has major drawbacks that are much less evident with benzodiazepines. Table 3-2 summarizes the characteristics of various benzodiazepine hypnotics.

Among the benzodiazepines, it is sometimes difficult to make choices. One tends to go with experience, so after many years of widespread clinical use and acceptance by patients, flurazepam may merit preference. For those patients who show daytime impairment seen with the lowest possible dose of this drug, one might consider a very short-acting drug, such as triazolam. Temazepam has no discernible advantages over other drugs with a short duration of action; lorazepam might be an alternative choice among this group. For occasional use, it is difficult to beat diazepam. The action of single doses is much shorter than the half-life would lead one to believe, as effects of such doses are quickly terminated by distribution. Rapid entry into the brain provides for a quick onset of action. Triazolam has become the favorite hypnotic and now accounts for the majority of sales. Temazepam and flurazepam have been relegated to lesser use.

The drug may act faster if it is given in liquid form, but most hypnotics are available only in tablet or capsule form. Taking fluid with the drug, to assure prompt disintegration and suspension of the material, may hasten absorption. Remaining active or upright for a short time after taking the medication may also enhance absorption. This can be accomplished to some degree by taking the dose about an hour before bedtime.

**Table 3-2. Characteristics of Benzodiazepine Hypnotics**

|            | Advantages   | Disadvantages   | Doses               |
|------------|--------------|-----------------|---------------------|
| Flurazepam | Long-acting  | May accumulate  | 15, 30 mg           |
| Temazepam  | Intermediate | Slow absorption | 15, 30 mg           |
| Triazolam  | Short-acting | ? rebound       | 0.25, 0.5, 1.0 mg   |

## Low Doses

The required dose to produce a hypnotic effect will vary considerably among persons. It is most appropriate to begin with the smallest possible doses and then increase them until the desired effect on insomnia is obtained with a minimal amount of daytime hangover. Many patients may respond well to a dose of 0.125 mg of triazolam (which one must obtain by breaking a 0.25 mg tablet). Unfortunately, it is not possible to obtain equivalent doses of temazepam or flurazepam, as these drugs come in fixed dose units that do not lend themselves to such manipulation.

Most authorities now feel that maximum doses should not be exceeded. The maximum for triazolam might be 0.5 mg, for flurazepam 60 mg, and for temazepam 60 mg. Patients who are unresponsive to doses of this magnitude must have developed some degree of cross-tolerance from use of other drugs or alcohol.

Many patients will note some hangover soon after awakening. If this sluggishness disappears after an hour or two of moving about, or after the morning cup of coffee, it is not of any great concern. One should be alert for more convincing evidences of daytime impairment: a continued feeling of lethargy, a tendency to fall asleep during the day, increased mistakes in performing familiar tasks, and such. Evidence of such daytime impairment must be construed as being due to a dose that was too large.

## Limited Duration of Use

Hypnotics should be used occasionally and not habitually. The patient must be told that insomnia does not seriously damage health; a night of poor sleep will probably be rectified the following night without any pharmacologic intervention. If this premise is accepted, one would use a hypnotic drug only after at least two consecutive nights of poor sleep. This practice alone should make their use intermittent and relatively infrequent. Patients should be told that after taking a single dose of a drug such as flurazepam, they may still have lingering effects the next night. Thus, taking two consecutive doses of a long-acting hypnotic is seldom necessary for the treatment of simple insomnia. However, some patients ignore this advice and use drugs regularly, often with little evidence of harm.

## NEW PHARMACOLOGIC APPROACHES

A substantial number of new benzodiazepines that may be marketed as hypnotics are in various phases of development or are sold in some countries. These include flunitrazepam (an intermediate-acting drug), midalozam (a very short-acting drug), quazepam and clobazam (long-acting drugs), brotizolam, and lormetazepam. It seems unlikely that any of these additional entries will offer any substantial advantage over those benzodiazepines currently available.

A comparison of two benzodiazepines, one with an intermediate elimination half-life (temazepam, 15 mg) and one with a long half-life (quazepam, 15 mg) showed that tolerance tended to develop to the efficacy of temazepam but quazepam had more hangover effects (Kales et al., 1986b). Lorazepam, a drug with a short to intermediate half-life, produced rebound anxiety and withdrawal following long-term use (Kales et al., 1986a). The problem with studies such as these is that they throw no light on the efficacy of these drugs if used as they should be, for limited times, and intermittently. None of the benzodiazepines is perfect. Whether any are better than others is doubtful.

A new class of hypnotics, represented by suriclone and zopiclone, are under investigation. Although these drugs are not benzodiazepines, they act by binding to benzodiazepine receptors. Whether or not they have an appreciable advantage over benzodiazepines is not clear.

L-tryptophan is still promoted as a "natural" hypnotic even though pharmacologic doses (usually more than 1 g given separately from food) are used. A controlled comparison with flurazepam favored the latter drug. Nightly doses of 3 g did not shorten sleep latency until the fourth night of treatment, hardly acceptable for someone wanting to go to sleep now (Spinweber, 1986). Its safety in long-term use is not established.

# ADVERSE EFFECTS

## Dependence

Benzodiazepines taken chronically have the potential of producing dependence. The likelihood of dependence is considerably reduced when these drugs are taken in small doses and infrequently. The long half-life of desalkylflurazepam probably protects against a severe withdrawal reaction. On the other hand, one might expect such reactions with a short-acting drug, such as triazolam. An isolated withdrawal seizure occurred 30 hours after the last dose in a patient who had taken 1.25 mg of the drug nightly for 2 weeks (Tien and Gujavarty, 1985). On the other hand, a more classic type of withdrawal syndrome and seizure was observed in a man who took doses of 7 to 10 mg/day of triazolam for self-management of anxiety (Schneider et al., 1987). Thus, it is possible to become dependent on benzodiazepine hypnotics, but it requires considerable misuse.

## Rebound Insomnia and Anxiety

Rebound anxiety and insomnia have been reported with short half-life drugs, such as triazolam, sometimes occurring late in the night's sleep as the drug effect wears off (Bixler et al., 1985). This concept has been somewhat controversial, being observed by some investigators but not by others. The phenomenon of drug withdrawal from a single dose has not been established before. One could imagine that insomnia the night following a dose of hypnotic may simply represent some degree of "over-sleeping," so that the main drive for sleep, its deprivation, is not as strong as usual. One would not become thirsty for some time after drinking 2 liters of fluid.

## Oversedation

Oversedation may be brought about by causes other than taking excessive doses of hypnotics. Many patients take daytime sedatives, tranquilizers, antihistamines, and other drugs that add to the residual effects of hypnotics. These actions may be unknown to patients or their physicians. Barbiturates, particularly, synergize with the respiratory depression caused by alcohol. This combination may lead to unexpected and unintended deaths.

Almost all hypnotic drugs have some type of hangover effects. Unwanted residual sedation from flurazepam was found in only 78 of 2542 hospitalized patients for whom it was prescribed. As might be expected, it was more prevalent with 30-mg doses than with 15-mg doses and was more common among older patients than those under age 60 years. If older patients were given the larger dose, the increase in residual sedation was dramatic (Greenblatt et al., 1977). One might infer that the long-acting metabolite of flurazepam is cleared even less well in older patients. To reiterate, the dose of hypnotic drug should be the least amount that will suffice: The smallest doses possible should always be tried first.

## Respiratory Depression

Benzodiazepines are much less likely than barbiturates to cause respiratory depression. This consideration becomes critical in patients with chronic obstructive pulmonary disease, who are often precipitated into acute respiratory failure by sedative drugs. Customary hypnotic doses of triazolam were found not to have adverse effects on respiration in patients without severe waking hypoxemia or carbon dioxide retention (Timms et al., 1988). Thus, it would appear that small doses of benzodiazepine hypnotics may be employed to remedy the disturbed sleep so many of these patients experience. However, sleep apnea is likely to be aggravated by any drug that may decrease respiratory drive. This condition is a relative contraindication to use of such drugs unless it has been alleviated by tracheostomy or some other surgical procedure.

## Amnesia

This side effect, which might have been anticipated, seems to be unusually common with triazolam. Patients have reported functioning for 24 hours or more following a hypnotic dose of the drug without any memory of this time period. What causes such severe anterograde amnesia is uncertain. Coincident use of alcohol has occurred in some cases, but not in others. Although triazolam was reported to produce a variety of bizarre psychological effects some years back after its introduction in the Netherlands, these reactions were clearly dose related. It has been more difficult to establish a clear dose relationship in the case of amnesia. Oddly enough, cases occurring in medical or scientific personnel traveling to professional meetings seem to be over-represented.

## Suicide

Hypnotic—sedative drugs are the chemical agents most commonly used for committing suicide. Because many patients with insomnia may have masked emotional disorders, the physician should try to minimize the danger of suicide by prescribing small total amounts at any time. The management of the consequences of overdose of these drugs is essentially the same as that for the antianxiety drugs reviewed in Chapter 2.

## REFERENCES

Bixler EO, Kales JD, Kales A, et al (1985) Rebound insomnia and elimination half-life: assessment of individual subject response. J Clin Pharmacol 25:115—124

Chase MH (1986) Overview of sleep research, Circa 1985. Sleep 9:452—457

Chweh AY, Lin YB, Swinyard EA (1984) Hypnotic action of benzodiazepines: a possible mechanism. Life Sci 34:1763—1768

Feinberg I, Fein G, Walker JM, et al (1979) Flurazepam effects on sleep EEG. Visual, computer and cycle analysis. Arch Gen Psychiatry 36:95—102

Greenblatt DJ, Abernethy DR, Divoll M, et al (1983) Pharmacokinetics properties of benzodiazepine hypnotics. J Clin Psychopharmacol 3:129—132

Greenblatt DJ, Allen MD, Shader RI (1977) Toxicity of high-dose flurazepam in the elderly. Clin Pharmacol Ther 21:355—361

Guilleminault C, Eldridge FL, Dement WC (1973) Insomnia with sleep apnea: a new syndrome. Science 181:856—858

Hauri P (1975) Insomnia and other sleep disorders. pp 11—24. In Kagan F, Harwood T, Rickels K, et al (eds): Hypnotics. Methods of Development and Evaluation. Spectrum, New York

Horne JA, Shackell BS (1987) Slow wave sleep elevations after body heating: proximity to sleep and effects of aspirin. Sleep 10:383—392

Jochemsen R, van Boxtel CJ, Hermans J, Breimer DD (1983) Kinetics of five benzodiazepine hypnotics in healthy subjects. Clin Pharmacol Ther 34:42—47

Jouvet M (1969) Biogenic amines and the state of sleep. Science 163:32—41

Kales A, Bixler EO, Soldatos CR, et al (1986a) Lorazepam: effects on sleep and withdrawal phenomena. Pharmacology 32:121—130

Kales A, Bixler EO, Soldatos CR, et al (1986b) Quazepam and temazepam: effects of short- and intermediate-term use and withdrawal. Clin Pharmacol Ther 39:345—352

Kales A, Malstrom EJ, Scharf MB, Rubin RT (1969) Psychological and biochemical changes following use and withdrawal of hypnotics. pp 331—343. In Kales A (ed): Sleep: Physiology and Pathology. *A Symposium.* JB Lippincott, Philadelphia

Krueger JM, Karaszewski JW, Davenne D, Shoham S (1986) Somnogenic muramyl peptides. Fed Proc 45:2552—2555

Meddis R (1977) The Sleep Instinct. Routledge and Kegan Paul, London

Mellinger GD, Balter MB, Uhlenhuth EH (1985) Insomnia and its treatment. Prevalence and correlates. Arch Gen Psychiatry 42:225—232

Miller LG, Greenblatt DJ, Abernethy DR, et al (1988) Kinetics, brain uptake, and receptor binding characteristics of flurazepam and its metabolites. Psychopharmacology 94:386–391

Moore-Ede MC, Czeisler CA, Richardson GS (1983) Circadian timekeeping in health and disease. N Engl J Med 309:469–536

NIH Consensus Conference (1984) Drugs and insomnia. The use of medication to promote sleep. JAMA 251:2410–2414

Parmeggiani PL (1987) Interaction between sleep and thermoregulation: an aspect of the control of behavioral states. Sleep 10:426–435

Schneider LS, Syapin P, Pawluczyk S (1987) Seizures following triazolam withdrawal despite benzodiazepine treatment. J Clin Psychiatry 48:418–419

Shader RI, Greenblatt DJ (1983) Triazolam and anterograde amnesia: all is not well in the Z-zone. J Clin Psychopharmacol 3:273

Spinweber CL (1986) l-Tryptophan administered to chronic sleep-onset insomniacs: late-appearing reduction of sleep latency. Psychopharmacology 90:151–155

Tien AY, Gujavarty KS (1985) Seizure following withdrawal from triazolam. Am J Psychiatry 142:1516–1517

Timms RM, Dawson A, Hajdukovic RM, Mitler MM (1988) Effect of triazolam on sleep and arterial oxygen saturation in patient with chronic obstructive pulmonary disease. Arch Intern Med 149:2159–2163

# 4

## ANTIDEPRESSANTS

### HISTORY

Soon after their introduction into medical practice in the late 1930s, amphetamines were used for treating depression. Over the years, these drugs were not considered to be very effective for the chronically and severely depressed patient, although they were sometimes helpful in milder, more acute depressions.

Iproniazid produced euphoria in patients with tuberculosis, in whom it was first used in 1952, but this observation lay dormant for several years. One reason was that several subsequent studies of depressed patients used isoniazid, which had been substituted for iproniazid. The assumption that isoniazid had the same pharmacologic activity as iproniazid, on which several negative reports of its efficacy were based, was soon negated by laboratory studies indicating that iproniazid was a much more potent inhibitor of the enzyme monoamine oxidase (MAO).

As early as 1954, reserpine was found to produce clinical depression, both in hypertensives as well as in normal persons. Its mechanism of action was soon defined as mediated by altering the storage of biogenic amines in nerve terminals, so new attention was paid to drugs that might increase biogenic amine concentrations in the brain. As MAO was an enzyme that catabolized these amines, use of an inhibitor seemed to be a reasonable way to effect this increase. Accordingly, renewed clinical studies of iproniazid were undertaken in 1956 which suggested that the hypothesis might be correct (Zeller, 1959).

Almost simultaneously, clinical investigations of a compound that seemed to be a minor structural variant of the phenothiazine, promazine, indicated that it was not a useful antipsychotic, as had been supposed, but that it might have antidepressant properties. This drug, imipramine, was soon established as a new type of antidepressant (Kuhn, 1958). Thus, by 1957, two new types of antidepressant drugs were available, the MAO inhibitors and the tricyclic antidepressants.

Both MAO inhibitors and tricyclics proliferated during the 1960s and 1970s. By the end of the 1970s, seven tricyclics and three MAO inhibitors were on the market in the United States, and there seemed to be little point in expanding these numbers. Beginning in the 1980s, newer classes of drugs have appeared. These have been lumped together as *second-generation antidepressants* or, because of their chemical diversity, termed *heterocyclics*. Four of these drugs, amoxapine, maprotiline, trazodone, and fluoxetine, have reached the marketplace and others are in the wings.

# CLINICAL ASPECTS OF DEPRESSION
## Prevalence

The same Epidemiologic Catchment Area (ECA) program that reported on the frequency of anxiety disorders (see Chapter 2) has made estimates of both the 6-month and lifetime prevalence rates of depressive disorders. The 6-month prevalence of major depressive disorder ranged from 2.2 to 3.5 percent and for minor depression, dysthymia, from 2.1 to 3.8 percent (Myers et al., 1984). The lifetime prevalence rates for major depression ranged between 3.7 to 6.7 percent and for dysthymia between 2.1 and 3.8 percent (Robins et al., 1984). Such prevalence rates are somewhat lower than previous estimates. Nonetheless, if only 400,000 persons annually are treated for depression, a huge number of patients may remain untreated and possibly unrecognized.

Although not all suicides are directly related to depression, a substantial number are. Suicide is the third leading cause of death among the age group of 15 to 34 years and the tenth leading cause of death among all ages. For every known suicide, there may be severalfold more "hidden" suicides. Thus, depression is not only frequent but it has an appreciable mortality rate in addition to its considerable morbidity.

## Diagnosis

Depression is readily diagnosed when it is the patient's chief complaint; unfortunately, it rarely is. A host of complaints may mask the true underlying disorder. Patients with many vague complaints, most or all of which defy explanation, and those who may be thought to be "neurotic" or "crocks" should be suspected of being depressed.

Depression and anxiety are inextricable. The initial complaints of depressed patients are often physical; some manifestations, such as fatigue, headache, insomnia, and gastrointestinal disturbances, resemble those of simple anxiety. Other complaints may be more distinctive, such as anorexia and weight loss, bad taste in the mouth, chronic pain, loss of interest, inactivity, loss of sexual desire, and a general feeling of despondency. The constellation of fatigue, musculoskeletal complaints, sleep disorder, and loss of joy in living is characteristic of depression. Guilt is a feeling almost unique to depression; if anger is directed toward rather than inward, hostility may predominate. The core depressive syndrome consists of somatic complaints, anxiety-tension, guilt, and various manifestations of a depressed mood.

As any empathetic physician must know, depression is a most uncomfortable disorder. A physician with a strong family history of depression, who suffered seasonal depressions, graphically described how bad such patients feel: ". . . bouts of insomnia, paranoid ideation and social withdrawal; . . . this illness hurts, with a deep and abiding pain . . . physical symptoms . . . well described (anorexia, constipation, fatigue) . . . some not so well known (arthralgias, paresthesias, headache); . . . isolation, the "crawl-in-a-hole" feeling; . . . inability to think clearly, to make even the simplest decisions; . . . general irritability and inability to tolerate social interaction; . . . racing thoughts, especially between 3 and 5 A.M. in which every terrible event of one's life flashes across the screen, precluding any form of sleep; . . . swept away by suicidal thoughts." (Butler, 1986). Our terrible lack in medicine is the inability to get inside the skin of our patients. We owe a great debt to our colleagues who are willing to share such experiences with us.

## Nosology of Depression

The nosology of depression has been marked by a tremendously confusing nomenclature of dichotomies: primary and secondary (somewhat related to the endogenous–reactive division); neurotic and psychotic (based on attendant behavioral symptoms); agitated and retarded (based on motor phenomena); and the recently introduced major–minor dichotomy (based on severity of illness). The recent revival of the terms *bipolar* and *unipolar* adds even more confusion; essentially, bipolar depressions are those associated with episodes of mania.

Be that as it may, both DSM-III and its minor revision separate "major depression" (which might previously have been called "endogenous") from "bipolar disorder" (which in a more reasonable nomenclature would retain the highly descriptive term, "manic-depressive disorder"). Both these categories are subserved by the recognition of minor forms of the illness, such as dysthymia and cyclothymic disorder. And then there are wastebaskets in which to put other cases that do not neatly fit these categories. It is really difficult to detect any new concepts in this new classification, which is primarily based on clinical manifestations regardless of possible etiology. Its advantage is that relatively well-defined diagnostic criteria are stated for each diagnosis. Thus, although we may not know much about what we are describing, we will at least all be talking about similar clinical situations.

## ETIOLOGIC CONSIDERATIONS

### Heterogeneity

The great variety of terms to describe depressions, as well as the many schemes for classifying them, strongly suggests that they are heterogeneous. Depression may be viewed as a symptom (all of us feel "depressed" from time to time), a syndrome (one may be depressed from losing one's job, losing a loved one, or having a serious illness), or as a disorder (some people become seriously depressed for little apparent reason).

Psychologically, most depressions involve a feeling of loss—of health, wealth, a loved one, self-esteem, or youthful vigor. One of the paradoxes of depression is that some patients who become depressed have all the outward trappings of success; their loss is their failure to meet self-imposed standards of excellence. The anger engendered by the loss may be directed inward, suicide being the most inwardly hostile action. Some psychological treatments are based on encouraging the outward expression of anger in depressed patients.

The model of depression produced by reserpine formed the basis for present-day concepts of the genetic-biochemical basis for depression. The following syllogism developed: Reserpine evoked depression; reserpine depleted storage of biogenic amines from synaptic vesicles; therefore, depression was associated with a deficiency of neurotransmission involving biogenic amines.

Thus, we have two possible etiologic bases for depressive illnesses. One emphasizes life experiences and implies that treatment should be psychosocial, that is, some sort of psychotherapy. The other implies that depressed persons have a biologic substrate that makes them unable to cope normally with the vicissitudes of life, so that stresses that might only evoke a minor, transient depressed state in a normal person provoke serious, lasting depression. Such an interactive model suggests that life experience may determine the time of onset, severity, and type of manifestations of the disorder, although the biochemical defect would constitute the necessary condition for its appearance.

## Amine Hypothesis

The amine hypothesis of depression is based largely on circumstantial evidence. First, the reserpine model of depression is associated with depletion of biogenic amines, principally norepinephrine and serotonin, but also dopamine. Second, drugs effective in treating depression have effects on these aminergic systems. Tricyclics block uptake mechanisms for both norepinephrine and serotonin; MAO inhibitors block the enzyme principally involved in their degradation. Sympathomimetics have a variety of actions, but in sum they also tend to increase the availability of these amine neurotransmitters at the synapse.

Direct proof of the amine hypothesis has been difficult. If deficient aminergic neurotransmission were of primary pathogenetic importance, one would expect that levels of their metabolites, 3-methoxy-4-hydroxy-phenylglycol (MHPG), in the case of norepinephrine, and 5-hydroxy-indoleacetic acid (5-HIAA), in the case of serotonin, would be decreased in depressed patients. Such evidence has been difficult to substantiate. To complicate matters further, treatment with imipramine and amitriptyline causes further significant decreases in these neurotransmitter metabolites (from 35 to 41 percent), which might be expected to make matters worse (Bowden et al., 1985). Furthermore, not all drugs that have been found to be clinically effective antidepressants block uptake mechanisms: iprindole, mianserin, and trazodone seem to work differently, although it must be noted that questions have been raised about their clinical efficacy.

## Receptor Hypotheses

For a long time, increased aminergic neurotransmitters in the synapse were thought to increase postsynaptic responses in a deficient system. Such conclusions were based on acute studies. Clinically, however, drugs are given chronically, which is necessary for their antidepressant action. When chronic administration is done in animals, and the consequences postsynaptically are measured by the generation of cyclic AMP, a subsensitivity of postsynaptic beta-adrenoreceptors is observed (Vetulani and Sulser, 1975). Thus, thinking about the consequences of increased aminergic neurotransmission from antidepressants has made a 180-degree turn. The implications are now strong that the original theory was incorrect.

During the past decade, attention has turned to the effects of various antidepressants on receptors rather than primarily on neurotransmitters, even though in some cases changes in receptors follow changes in neurotransmitters. Some of the many actions of antidepressants on various receptor systems are summarized in Table 4-1. Most work has focused on the norepinephrine-receptor-coupled adenylate cyclase system. Most drugs with antidepressant actions, as well as such nondrug treatments as electroconvulsive therapy (ECT) or sleep deprivation, cause subsensitivity of this system with down-regulation of the number of beta-adrenoreceptors. However, an intact serotonergic system is required for down-regulation of beta-receptors to occur. These findings have suggested a link between the two neurotransmitter systems and their receptors (Sulser, 1987). Thus, the previous controversy about the relative

**Table 4-1.** Actions of Tricyclic and Other Antidepressants on Receptors

| Agent | Actions |
| --- | --- |
| Beta-2-adrenoreceptor | Down-regulation due to increased presence of agonist, norepinephrine |
| 5-HT-2 receptor | Down-regulation due to increased presence of agonist, serotonin |
| 5-HT—1A receptor | Down-regulation; effect uncertain |
| Alpha-2-adrenoreceptor | Down-regulation of inhibition by this receptor presynaptically leading to increased release of norepinephrine |
| Alpha-1-adrenoreceptor | Blocked, producing hypotension and sedation |
| Muscarinic acetylcholine receptors | Antagonized; anticholinergic effects; sedation; questionable pertinence to antidepressant effects |
| Histamine H-1 receptors | Antagonized; producing sedation, ? antidepressant action |
| Histamine H-2 receptors | Antagonized, ? consequences |
| Dopamine receptor | Necessary for action of sympathomimetics, nomifensine, buproprion |
| GABA B receptor | Increased inhibition of serotonin release |

importance of serotonin and norepinephrine has been resolved by suggesting that they are mutually interdependent.

Some antidepressant drugs do not work on the NE-sensitive adenylate cyclase system, such as trazodone, trimipramine, and fluoxetine. These drugs may work more directly on serotonergic systems. Other drugs, such as buproprion, may act primarily through an effect on dopamine, although the role of this neurotransmitter and its receptors in depression is still uncertain. Alpha-2-adrenoreceptor blockade accentuates the down-regulation of beta-adrenoreceptors produced by tricyclics. Thus, specific alpha-2 antagonists may be useful as antidepressants, possibly in combination with others (Stahl and Palazidou, 1986).

Other receptors that may have a role to play in the drug treatment of depression include the 5HT–1A receptor, which becomes subsensitive following treatment with both antidepressants and ECT, as well as the GABA B receptor, which is increased following such treatment; the effect would be to increase its inhibition of the release of serotonin (Green, 1987).

The action of MAO inhibitors is consistent with the amine hypothesis. Presumably by reducing the catabolism of aminergic neurotransmitters (what might be construed as the "off-switch" of such transmission), they increase the action of neurotransmitters at the synapse. An anticipated secondary effect would be the down-regulation of the respective postsynaptic receptors.

## Other Possibilities for Pathogenesis or Modes of Drug Action

Many basic bodily rhythms, such as those of sleep, appetite, sexual desire, and motor activity, are disturbed in endogenous depressions. These observations have led to the hypothesis that the proximate precipitant of depression is due to some alteration in diurnal rhythms. Attempts to treat depression by altering these rhythms, such as by sleep deprivation or by advancing the phase of sleep–wake cycles, have only been partially successful because of practical considerations. Of course, it may still turn out that the ultimate cause of these disturbed rhythms may be due to disturbances in aminergic neurotransmission. On the other hand, REM sleep deprivation has been proposed as a mechanism of action of antidepressants (Vogel, 1983).

The apposition of adrenergic nerve fiber varicosities and cerebral capillaries has suggested that adrenergic control of the cerebral microcirculation by alpha-1-adrenoreceptor blockade from antidepressants should increase capillary permeability. Such changes have been observed with concentrations of tricyclic antidepressants close to therapeutic ranges. Furthermore, they require chronic treatment to attain their maximum effects, similar to the delay in clinical response to treatment. Tetrabenazine produces depression in animals as well as decreasing the responsiveness of cerebral blood flow to $CO_2$ exposure and the permeability of capillaries. These changes are ameliorated in a dose-dependent fashion by amitriptyline (Kent et al., 1986). Although this mechanism could be relevant to the action of tricyclics, it may be less relevant to the action of other antidepressants that have little or no alpha-1-receptor blocking action.

## Biologic Correlates of Depression

A diagnostic test that would confirm the clinical diagnosis of depression and be useful in planning drug therapy would be most welcome. A great deal of enthusiasm developed in the 1970s for measurement of urinary excretion of MHPG, a norepinephrine metabolite. If low excretion indicated a primary deficiency of norepinephrine and high excretion deficiency of serotonin, one might have a simple way to select the proper drug for individual patients based on the presumed biochemical defect. The only problem is that high and low levels in patients are precisely the same as they are in normals (Hollister et al., 1978). No precedent in all of medicine exists for making diagnostic or prognostic inferences based on variations within the normal range of a laboratory test. Although a number of studies indicated some utility of such measurement in predicting the clinical response to drugs, a more recent study concluded that the association between response to imipramine or desipramine and rate of MHPG excretion was so weak that predicting the clinical response to drugs based on this test would be premature (Muscettola et al., 1984).

A blunted response of pituitary thyrotropin (TSH) to thyrotropin-releasing hormone (TRH) has been repeatedly confirmed in about 25 to 35 percent of depressed patients. The meaning of this abnormality is totally unclear, but it may be dependent on prevailing levels of either growth hormone or cortisol. Although a blunted response, if it could be interpreted at all, might suggest a subclinical degree of hyperthyroidism, an exaggerated response, even in the presence of normal baseline TSH levels, has been construed as what might be called "sub-subclinical hypothyroidism" and interpreted as an indication for thyroidal supplements. This hypothesis has not yet been tested.

The dexamethasone suppression test, a variant of the one so useful in diagnosing hyperadrenocorticalism, has had a checkered history in psychiatry. It has been averred that nonsuppression augurs a better response to drug therapy and that reversion of the test to normal may indicate the end of a depressive episode, but clinical use of the test has been disappointing. First, many artifacts can influence the test, such as the bioavailability of the orally administered dexamethasone, variations in reliability of cortisol assays, and influences of age, weight, and other drugs (Nierenberg and Feinstein, 1988). Second, even when the test is used under the best possible circumstances, it is of little help in making diagnostic distinctions. Nonsuppression was common in manics, was similar in unipolar and bipolar depressed patients, and was unexpectedly frequent in normals (Stokes et al., 1984). Others have also found nonsuppression in patients with alcoholism and Alzheimer's disease. Thus, it would now appear that use of this test for making any inferences about use of antidepressants, either their selection or the duration of treatment, is unwarranted.

Another fairly consistent finding in depressed patients is that the first epoch of

REM sleep appears earlier in the night than normal. This reduced REM latency may be related to the changes in diurnal rhythms mentioned earlier. Although it has been more consistent than other tests in reflecting depression, it is seldom used as a diagnostic test because of the complexity of such studies.

The significance of these various biologic correlates of depression is unclear. Are they related in some way to the pathogenesis of depression or are they epiphenomena? The fact that many of these abnormalities revert to normal with remission of depression suggests that they may represent state rather than trait characteristics. Furthermore, correlations between the various markers are not particularly strong (Davis et al., 1981).

# TYPES OF ANTIDEPRESSANTS

The number of drugs available for treating depression has been growing rapidly. The original group was exemplified by the tricyclic antidepressants, the MAO inhibitors, and, to a lesser extent, the sympathomimetic amines and lithium. This group might be referred to as *first-generation antidepressants*. During the past several years, a number of other drugs, usually chemically and sometimes pharmacologically different from these other classes, have been introduced. These drugs are often called *second-generation antidepressants*.

## Tricyclics

Chemical structures of some of the most commonly used tricyclics are shown in Figure 4-1. Slight modifications occur in either the ring structure or side chain. Even though slight, these chemical alterations provide pharmacologic differences among the various tricyclics.

### Imipramine

This drug was the first antidepressant, discovered fortuitously in the clinic. The major metabolic pathway is demethylation, which leads to formation of desipramine, an active metabolite. The amount of desipramine in steady-state conditions actually exceeds that of the parent compound in most patients.

An attempt to correlate plasma concentrations of imipramine: desipramine with clinical responses indicated that a 3 : 2 ratio of desipramine to imipramine was most favorable and that patients with ratios more than 5 : 2 or less than 1 : 1 were nonresponders. Such ratios are individual characteristics of patients and might be used to prognosticate clinical response early on in treatment (Rigal et al., 1987). Desipramine may be further oxidized to active metabolites, but the extent of their contribution to therapeutic effects is uncertain (Sutfin et al., 1984). Imipramine blocks the amine pump both for norepinephrine and serotonin; desipramine specifically blocks uptake of norepinephrine. The net effect is that imipramine blocks uptake of norepinephrine more than of

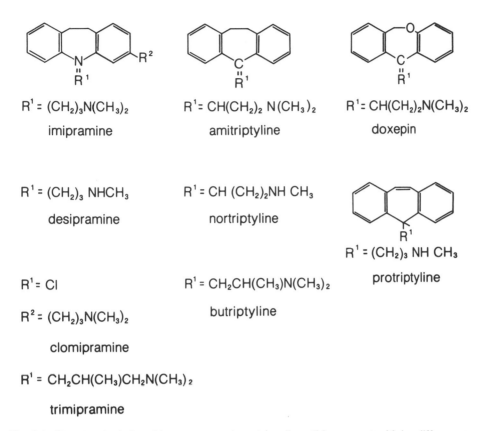

R$^1$ = (CH$_2$)$_3$N(CH$_3$)$_2$

imipramine

R$^1$= CH(CH$_2$)$_2$ N(CH$_3$)$_2$

amitriptyline

R$^1$= CH(CH$_2$)$_2$N(CH$_3$)$_2$

doxepin

R$^1$ = (CH$_2$)$_3$ NHCH$_3$

desipramine

R$^1$ = CH (CH$_2$)$_2$NH CH$_3$

nortriptyline

R$^1$ = (CH$_2$)$_3$ NH CH$_3$

protriptyline

R$^1$= Cl

R$^2$= (CH$_2$)$_3$N(CH$_3$)$_2$

clomipramine

R$^1$ = CH$_2$CH(CH$_3$)N(CH$_3$)$_2$

butriptyline

R$^1$ = CH$_2$CH(CH$_3$)CH$_2$N(CH$_3$)$_2$

trimipramine

**Fig. 4-1.** Structural relationships among various tricyclic antidepressants. Major differences are in minor changes in the ring or side chain.

serotonin. Moderate sedative and anticholinergic effects may be troublesome to some patients. Alpha-adrenoreceptor blocking actions may be greater than those of most other tricyclics, which predisposes to orthostatic hypotension. Imipramine is a membrane-active local anesthetic (as are other tricyclics), which gives it both antiarrhythmic and arrhythmogenic actions. Usual doses of the drug are 75 to 300 mg/day.

## Desipramine

A metabolite of imipramine, this drug is used as a separate entity. A quicker onset of action than the parent drug was postulated, but that contention has been difficult to prove. Desipramine has fewer sedative, anticholinergic, and alpha-adrenoreceptor blocking actions than most other tricyclics. Patients who cannot tolerate the unwanted effects produced by these pharmacologic actions may tolerate desipramine better. Doses are similar to those for imipramine.

## Amitriptyline

This tricyclic was the most widely used until recently. A demethylated metabolite, nortriptyline, is generally not as abundant as the parent drug. Although amitriptyline in vitro has a selective action in blocking uptake of serotonin, nortriptyline has a mixed action. The net result is that amitriptyline has a mixed effect, predominantly on serotonin.

As interesting concept, *reciprocal clearance,* has been proposed as a way of predicting outcome to treatment with amitriptyline. The ratio of plasma concentrations of amitriptyline plus nortriptyline divided by the daily dose of amitriptyline in milligrams (which is usually greater than 1.0) is used to predict outcome. The higher the ratio, the better the ultimate outcome (Burch et al., 1988).

Amitriptyline is probably the most sedative and most anticholinergic of all tricyclics; it is often used when sedation is desired. Doses are usually 75 to 300 mg/day.

## Nortriptyline

A metabolite of amitriptyline, this drug is also used as a separate entity. During the first pass through the liver, it is extensively metabolized to 10-hydroxy-nortriptyline, which is far more abundant than the parent compound. The exact amount of activity contributed by the metabolite is unknown. Biochemical studies indicate that nortriptyline has effects on noradrenergic, serotonergic, and dopaminergic systems and that the 10-hydroxy metabolite is probably more selective for noradrenergic neurons than the parent drug (Nordin et al., 1987). Relatively fewer sedative and anticholinergic actions occur with nortriptyline than with amitriptyline. Doses of nortriptyline have usually been lower than for the other tricyclics, although the basis of such conservatism has not been established.

## Doxepin

The strong sedative effects of this drug have been the basis for its promotion as an antianxiety as well as an antidepressant drug. A demethylated metabolite also contributes to its action. Doxepin itself has a relatively weak action in blocking the amine pump, despite the fact that it is generally thought to be equally effective as an antidepressant. Doses are similar to those of other tricyclics.

## Protriptyline

This drug has been one of the least popular tricyclics and has not been widely promoted. Some clinicians believe that it has a stimulating action; it is certainly the least sedative tricyclic. Some anticholinergic action remains. Protriptyline may be a reasonable alternative for patients who become overly sedated by the other tricyclics. Doses are considerably lower than those of other tricyclics, generally 10 to 40 mg/day.

## Others

Butriptyline and trimipramine are isobutyl side-chain modifications of amitriptyline and imipramine, respectively. They differ little from the prototype drugs. Clomipramine is a chlorinated ring-substituted homolog of imipramine. Just why this modification provides a presumed specific efficacy for obsessive-compulsive patients is unclear (see Chapter 2). Doses of these drugs are similar to those of other tricyclics.

## Monoamine Oxidase Inhibitors

MAO inhibitors are classified as hydrazides (−C−N−N-configuration) and nonhydrazides. The structures of some MAO inhibitors are shown in Figure 4-2.

### Phenelzine

This drug has been the most durable MAO inhibitor and is the only one currently promoted in the United States. Because early studies had cast some doubt about efficacy (possibly owing to inadequate doses) and because of fear of serious adverse reactions, MAO inhibitors languished for many years. During the past decade, they have become more popular. Phenelzine was as effective as imipramine in 32 patients with major depression and was superior to imipramine in 32 patients with dysthymic disorder (Vallejo et al., 1987). Atypical depressions (the definitions change frequently) characterized by having a mood reactive to situations, hyperphagia, hypersomnolence, leaden feeling, and sensitivity to rejection, responded better to phenelzine than to placebo or to imipramine (Quitkin et al., 1988). Thus it appears that MAO inhibitors have selected areas in which they may excel. It has long been known to clinicians that some depressed patients seem to respond specifically to MAO inhibitors.

At least 80 percent inhibition of MAO must be obtained for optimal clinical effects. Doses of 1 mg/kg/day are usually necessary to obtain such inhibition, but the process takes time and so does the regeneration of the enzyme. Improvement in patients may not be evident until 2 or more weeks of treatment. When the

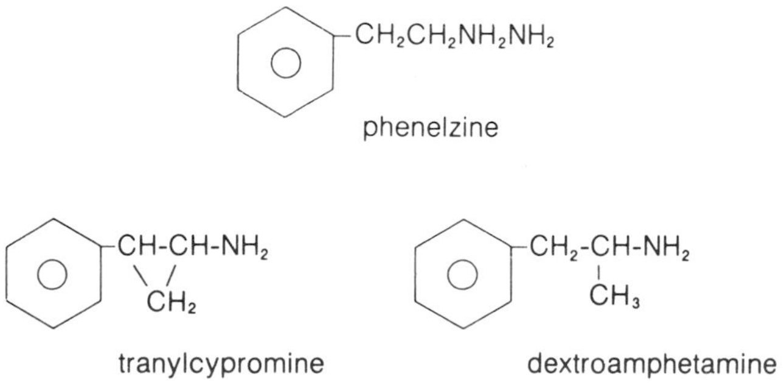

Fig. 4-2. MAO Inhibitors. Phenelzine is a hydrazide derivative (−C−N−N-configuration). Tranylcypromine is the cyclopropyl homolog of dextroamphetamine.

drug is stopped, the enzyme is not regenerated for another 2 weeks. Tricyclics should not be added or replaced in the treatment program for at least that period. The converse sequence of the MAO inhibitor following tricyclics can usually be done with no delay. Usual doses of phenelzine are 45 to 90 mg/day (Robinson et al., 1978).

## Isocarboxazid

This MAO inhibitor is neither widely used nor promoted and has been less well studied than the others. A recent evaluation of isocarboxazid compared it with placebo in 130 anxious depressives. The drug was more effective in several areas, including patients with major depression and those with atypical depression and reversed vegetative symptoms. It, too, seems to be effective in groups similar to those documented for phenelzine (Davidson et al., 1988). Usual doses are 20 to 50 mg/day.

## Tranylcypromine

The chemical structure of this nonhydrazide MAO inhibitor is similar to that of dextroamphetamine. It retains some of the sympathomimetic actions of the latter drug but is a much more potent inhibitor of MAO. Usual doses are 10 to 30 mg/day.

# Sympathomimetics

These drugs are used only in rare patients. Occasionally, they produce beneficial results in patients who have been resistant to the other antidepressants.

## Dextroamphetamine

The structure of this compound is shown in Figure 4-2. Insomnia and loss of appetite limit its use in some patients, although stimulation and appetite suppression may be desirable effects for others. Some patients require substantial doses to obtain benefit but show little evidence of tolerance or dependence with prolonged treatment. Usual doses are 10 to 30 mg/day, with some patients requiring as much as 60 mg/day. Methylphenidate, an amphetamine surrogate, is even less commonly used and has no special advantages.

# Lithium

Although lithium carbonate has been reported to be useful for treating acute depressions that appear not to be part of manic-depressive disorder, it is seldom used as a sole treatment. More likely it may be added to a tricyclic when the latter provides inadequate remission (De Montigny et al., 1981). Its use in preventing recurrences of depression, whether unipolar (endogenous) or bipolar (associated with manic episodes) is well documented. However, in a unipolar patient who has responded to a conventional antidepressant, it is usually easier to continue or maintain the patient on that drug than it is to switch to lithium.

# Second-Generation Antidepressants

The enthusiasm with which second-generation antidepressants have been received stems from the several problems that remain with the first-generation drugs. First, only about 60 to 65 percent of depressed patients are helped by first-generation drugs, and many do not attain a full remission of symptoms. Second, the clinical response to first-generation drugs may be delayed. This delay may be more a consequence of the slow induction of treatment mandated by the side effects of these drugs. Thus, it is more likely a pharmacokinetic than a pharmacodynamic phenomenon. Third, the numerous side effects of first-generation antidepressants may make it impossible to treat some patients with fully effective doses or may lead to noncompliance with treatment on the part of others. Finally, tricyclics in particular are potentially lethal when taken in overdose. The paradox is that one must prescribe such drugs to a group of patients with the highest risk of suicide.

Although it has not been claimed that the newer antidepressants are more effective overall than the tricyclics with which they are usually compared, they do assert three advantages: (1) a more rapid onset of action, (2) more tolerable side effects, (3) greater safety when taken in overdose (Coccaro and Siever, 1985).

Four of these drugs are currently on the market in the United States and more are expected soon. The variety of chemical structures of these drugs is shown in Figure 4-3.

## Amoxapine

Amoxapine is a demethylated metabolite of the antipsychotic loxapine. It is further metabolized to hydroxy metabolites, which are 3 to 10 times as abundant as the parent drug and which probably account for the antidepressant activity (Jue et al., 1982). The net effect is more blockade of uptake of norepinephrine than of serotonin. The anticholinergic action is weak. The dopamine-receptor blocking action of loxapine is retained to a somewhat lesser degree in amoxapine, which also has some antipsychotic activity. This combined action may be especially suitable for patients with psychotic or agitated depressions. However, it may also lead to extrapyramidal syndromes and hyperprolactinemia with sexual disturbances in men and amenorrhea-galactorrhea in women. Although the drug has less cardiotoxic action than tricyclics in overdoses, it produces seizures that are difficult to control, with an attendant fatality rate. Usual doses are 150 to 300 mg/day.

The claim for a more rapid onset of action is not substantiated and is further offset by an apparent tolerance to the therapeutic effects that may develop in some patients after an initial response. Not only are the usual sedative and anticholinergic side effects of tricyclics as common with this drug, but it also adds some of the side effects of antipsychotics. Severe neurotoxicity, which occurs after overdoses, makes it at least as dangerous as those tricyclics with predominant cardiotoxicity. In summary, amoxapine offers very little.

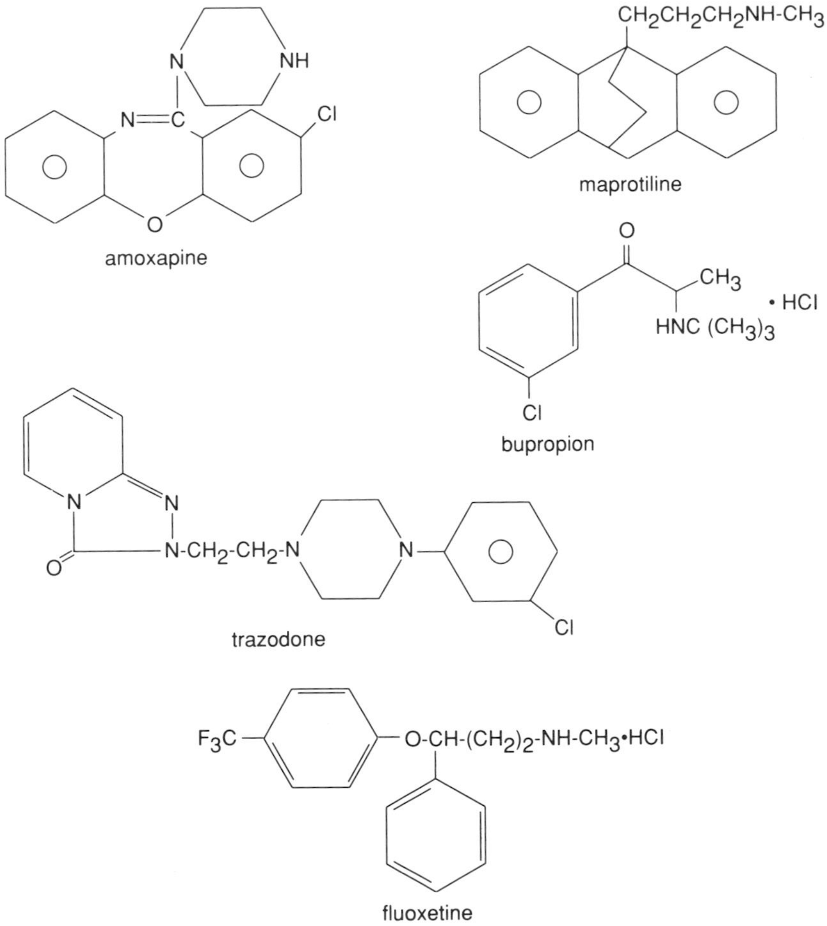

**Fig. 4-3.** Structures of second-generation antidepressants. A variety of structures are involved.

## Maprotiline

A two-carbon bridge across the central ring of the 6-6-6 three-ring structure of this drug creates a fourth ring, making it a tetracyclic compound. The side chain is the same monodemethylated aminopropyl side chain found in desipramine, creating a rather similar structural geometry. The primary action of the drug is to block uptake of norepinephrine; it also has less sedative or anticholinergic action than amitriptyline, the drug to which it has most often been compared. An unusual pharmacologic action of the drug has been to decrease the apparent number of benzodiazepine/beta-carboline recognition sites, possibly by inducing the production of some endogenous peptide ligand (Barbaccia et al., 1986). The clinical implications are uncertain.

The drug had a decade of use in other countries before arriving in the United

States and was well recognized to cause seizures, even within the range of therapeutic doses. Most seizures were dose related, which has led to a downward revision of recommended doses. The former range was 100 to 300 mg/day. Now it is believed that during the first 6 weeks of treatment, the maximum dose should be no more than 225 mg/day and that maintenance doses be no more than 200 mg/day. The drug should be used with care in combination with other drugs that may lower seizure thresholds and probably not be used at all in patients with abnormal electroencephalograms (Dessain et al., 1986).

Whether maprotiline has a faster onset of action has not been adequately tested. It seems to offer nothing new in its mechanism of action nor fewer sedative and anticholinergic side effects as compared with desipramine. Seizures occur at therapeutic doses far more often than with tricyclics. Rashes also seem to be more frequent. Overdoses are about as dangerous as with tricyclics. The drug offers little advantage over desipramine. Oxaprotiline, an active metabolite, is under clinical investigation but should not be much different.

## Trazodone

Although frequently described as a triazolopyridine compound, trazodone is more properly described as a phenylpiperazine. In this respect it chemically resembles oxypertine, a drug that has been used both as an antipsychotic and as an antianxiety agent. Pharmacologically, it is complicated (Silvestrini and Valeri, 1984). At some doses it acts as a serotonin receptor antagonist, whereas at others it acts both as a serotonin agonist and as an uptake inhibitor. It may also increase release of norepinephrine by blocking alpha-2 adrenoreceptors. The exact mode of its therapeutic action is unknown, although presumably it works mainly as a serotonergic drug. An active metabolite, *m*-chlorophenylpiperazine, is formed; whether or not it enhances or inhibits the action of trazodone is not clear; in one study it inhibited at least one action of trazodone (Vetulani et al., 1984).

Most clinical trials have compared the drug with existing tricyclic antidepressants, such as imipramine and amitriptyline. In general, it has been comparable to these standard agents, with few anticholinergic or cardiovascular side effects (Feighner and Boyer, 1988). In clinical practice, however, results have often been spotty. Some patients obtain much relief; others derive no benefit. The same dichotomy applies to its sedative effects. These side effects limit doses in some patients; others are not at all bothered. The spotty clinical responses have even led some investigators to question whether the drug should be used in endogenous depressions (Klein and Muller, 1985). The usual daily doses are 150 to 400 mg.

No claim is made for a more rapid onset of action, which is difficult to prove at best. The anticholinergic side effects of tricyclics are definitely fewer with this drug, but sedation can be troublesome. Adverse reactions include drowsiness, dizziness, headache, nausea, and priapism (Warner et al., 1987). The last-named may be heralded by spontaneous erections without obvious cause. A few instances of ventricular tachycardia have been reported, although this arrhythmia does not seem to be a problem when overdoses are taken

(Aronson and Hafez, 1986). Overdoses are generally easily managed and rarely fatal. The relative lack of side effects as well as the safety of the drug in overdose have made trazodone a huge commercial success. Questions do linger about its efficacy, however.

## Buproprion

Buproprion has a phenethylamine structure that superficially resembles that of amphetamine or methoxamine. Chemical modifications on the ring and side chain have markedly changed its spectrum of pharmacologic actions. The chlorine atom on the ring protects against rapid metabolism; the tertiary alkyl group is not readily dealkylated, avoiding pressor activity; the aminoketo group confers lipid solubility (Soroko et al., 1977).

The exact mode of action of buproprion is unclear. It definitely seems to require the presence of intact dopamine neurons in the brain. An early study suggested that the drug acted primarily as a dopamine uptake inhibitor (Cooper et al., 1980). It has little effect on norepinephrine uptake, no anticholinergic actions, and no inhibiting effects on monoamine oxidase. Long-term treatment produced neither down-regulation of beta-adrenoreceptors nor of dopamine receptors. It is possible that its major pharmacologic effects may be mediated by an active metabolite.

Dry mouth is the most common side effect. Rashes may occur in 1 to 2 percent of patients. Anorexia and mild agitation may also be observed. Seizures have occurred with high doses even within the presumed therapeutic range of doses (450 mg or more). For this reason, the drug was temporarily withdrawn from medical practice soon after it was approved. Recently, it has been re-introduced for use at generally lower doses than those previously used.

A more rapid onset of action than that of conventional antidepressants has not been documented. The drug also lacks most of the sedative, anticholinergic, and cardiovascular side effects of tricyclic antidepressants, although it is equally effective. Overdoses of from 900 to 3000 mg have been easily managed without any cardiovascular problems. Thus, the drug could offer significant advantages if the problem with seizures is avoided by lower doses.

## Fluoxetine

Fluoxetine is the first entirely specific serotonin uptake inhibitor. Not only is this property of interest, but it should allow testing of hypotheses about the relative importance of serotonin and norepinephrine in depression. It has little or no action on other neurotransmitters or receptors, which affords a specificity of action that may reduce unwanted effects. The drug has an active metabolite, norfluoxetine, which has similar pharmacologic actions. Both fluoxetine and its metabolite have very long plasma half-lives, from 1 to 3 days in the case of fluoxetine (4 days following chronic administration) to 7 days for the metabolite. Like other antidepressants, even those without a direct action on norepinephrine, fluoxetine causes decreased beta-adrenergic receptors in brain following chronic administration (Byerly et al., 1988).

A number of comparisons with placebo, amitriptyline, imipramine, and doxepin have shown the drug to be superior to placebo and equivalent to the standard drugs (Schatzberg et al., 1987). The usual range of doses have been 20 to 80 mg/day, although 20 to 40 mg/day may be adequate for most patients. The most common side effects are nausea, anorexia, diarrhea, anxiety, jitteriness, insomnia, and headache.

Fluvoxamine, which, despite its similar sounding name, is quite different in chemical structure, is another specific serotonin uptake inhibitor currently being developed for clinical use (Benfield and Ward, 1986).

## Benzodiazepines: Alprazolam

Various reports have suggested that benzodiazepines, such as diazepam, may be effective in some patients with depression characterized by much anxiety (Hollister et al., 1971). These types of depressions would generally be considered nonendogenous. A triazolobenzodiazepine, alprazolam, exhibits the same profile of pharmacologic activities as most other benzodiazepines (Rudzik et al., 1973). These actions would certainly justify its use as an antianxiety drug but do not explain why it should be different from other benzodiazepines in being an effective antidepressant. The efficacy of the drug in depression rests largely on a multiclinic trial that compared alprazolam (159 patients) with imipramine (146 patients) and placebo (131 patients). These patients met the standard research diagnostic criteria for depression. After 42 days of treatment, both active drugs produced more improvement in depression than placebo but were not different overall. Drowsiness was more often found in alprazolam-treated patients and dry mouth in those treated with imipramine (Feighner et al., 1983). Although the drug is not officially labeled for use as an antidepressant, many clinicians are prescribing it. Clinical consensus at the moment is that the drug may be useful in mildly depressed patients who are outpatients but that it is not fully effective in severe depressives.

About the only side effects that have been noted with alprazolam relate to its action on the central nervous system. Drowsiness has been the most common complaint. Yet even the frequency and intensity of this side effect seem to be less than from comparable doses of other benzodiazepines. Some of the studies of the drug in depressed patients have used doses up to 10 mg/day (equivalent perhaps to 100 mg/day of diazepam). Thus, it is possible that should patients being treated with such doses be suddenly withdrawn from the drug, an abstinence syndrome would follow.

## Other New Drugs

Selective and reversible MAO inhibitors are currently under development. Two forms of the enzyme MAO have been found in brain. MAO-A preferentially uses serotonin and tyramine as substrates, whereas MAO-B uses phenethylamine and benzylamine. Norepinephrine and dopamine are equal substrates for both forms of the enzyme. The goal of research has been to attain selective

MAO-A and MAO-B inhibitors. Although selectivity may be shown pharmaco-logically in small doses, larger doses such as might be used clinically show less. A clinical trial of the presumably selective MAO-B inhibitor 1-deprenyl (selegiline) indicated that it was clearly superior to placebo. The doses used, 30 mg/day, are about where selectivity seems to be lost. Side effects were no more common than with placebo (Mann et al., 1989).

Another approach has been to develop reversible MAO inhibitors, as the current ones are irreversible, inhibiting the enzyme for as long as 2 weeks. The advantages of reversible inhibitors are many: (1) reversal of tyramine poten-tiation and the hypertensive crises associated with it; (2) safer combination therapy with tricyclics; (3) closer relationship between MAO inhibition and plasma concentrations of the drugs; (4) minimal effect on drug-metabolizing enzymes that may cause unfavorable interactions with other drugs (Benedetti and Dostert, 1985).

# PHARMACOKINETICS

Pharmacokinetic parameters of various antidepressants are summarized in Table 4-2.

Bioavailability is variable, and may be low in some patients and with some drugs. This variability has led to recommendations for monitoring of plasma concentrations of these drugs, although clinical responses might be an even better indicator of the availability of the drug. Protein-binding is high, but variations in binding, although they may suggest wide variations in clinical effects, do not seem to have created many clinical problems. Plasma half-life is usually around 24 hours with most tricyclics, but is conspicuously longer with protriptyline and fluoxetine. The latter drug may take a while to attain steady-state plasma concentrations. On the other hand, half-life is shortest with trazodone, which suggests that doses of this drug should always be divided. Most antidepressants have active metabolites, but the contribution of these metabolites to the clinical effect is questionable with some. As all these drugs are highly lipid-soluble, the volumes of distribution are huge. Thus, it would be unrealistic to try to rid the body of any of these drugs by dialysis when they have been taken in overdose. Therapeutic ranges of plasma concentrations have been described for many of these drugs. However, it should be remembered that for every study that has found a relationship between drug levels and clinical response, others have failed. At best, one can use these numbers only as guides.

MAO inhibitors are "hit-and-run" drugs that produce an "irreversible" inhibition of MAO that persists after the drug is gone. In general, it has been more productive to measure the inhibition of this enzyme in platelets than to measure plasma concentrations of these agents. Present feeling is that optimal antidepressant effects from these drugs require about 60 to 80 percent inhibition of the enzyme, a degree of inhibition attained with doses of approximately 1 mg/kg/day of phenelzine (Davidson et al., 1978).

# CLINICAL USE

## General Considerations

Several considerations affect the use of antidepressants. The greatest error is simply to misdiagnose depression. Because of the wide variety of symptomatic complaints of depressed patients, one may miss the diagnosis unless a high level of awareness of its possibility is maintained. The most common error is to misdiagnose a depressed patient as having an anxiety disorder, as anxiety is virtually an inevitable accompaniment of depression. Other disorders, such as grief, schizophrenia, or even dementia, may also be mistaken for depression. Antidepressants will not improve such conditions but may actually worsen symptoms.

Having considered the diagnosis and confirmed it, one must refine the problem further. What causes other than the interaction between genetic and psychosocial factors may have precipitated this episode of depression? Is the patient severely ill enough to merit treatment as an inpatient under a psychiatrist's care, or could a primary care physician undertake treatment under conditions of outpatient care? What is the risk of suicide and the urgency of treatment?

Determination of suicidal risk in individual patients is extremely difficult, if not impossible (Pokorny, 1983). It is far better to overdiagnose the possibility of suicide than to underestimate it.

The natural history of the disorder in a specific patient will have a bearing on treatment. Has the patient had previous episodes of depression? How were they manifested? How long did they last? Many severe depressions run a characteristic course of several months with apparent spontaneous remission. Where in such a course is the patient at present? What are the goals of treatment?—for the present episode?—for the long run? What sort of treatment is best—psychological treatment, antidepressant drugs, both, or an immediate course of ECT with drugs?

## Indications

The major indication for antidepressants is to treat depression, but a number of other indications have been established by clinical experience.

### Depression

These drugs are indicated for treating depressions, their major use. This indication has been kept broad deliberately, as it is presently unclear whether specific drugs or classes of drugs are preferred for one type of depression or another.

### Enuresis

Enuresis is another established indication for tricyclics. Proof of efficacy for this indication is substantial, but drug therapy is not the preferred approach to

**Table 4-2.** Pharmacokinetic Parameters of Various Antidepressants

| Drug | Bioavailability (%) | Protein Binding (%) | Plasma Half-life (h) | Metabolites in Plasma | Volume of Distribution (L/kg) | Therapeutic Plasma Concentrations (ng/ml) |
|---|---|---|---|---|---|---|
| Imipramine | 29–77 | 88–93 | 6–20 | Desipramine usually more; active | 20–30 | > 180 total |
| Amitriptyline | 31–61 | 82–96 | 19–31 | Nortriptyline; usually less, active | 15 | > 200 total |
| Desipramine | — | 70–90 | 14–30 | 2-Hydroxy metabolite | 22 | 145 |
| Nortriptyline | 46–79 | 93 | 18–28 | 10-Hydroxy; 3 to 4 times as abundant; ? activity | 21–57 | 50–150 |
| Doxepin | 13–45 | — | 8–24 | Desmethyl; active | 9–33 | — |
| Protriptyline | — | — | 55–124 | None active | 19–26 | 70–170 |
| Clomipramine | — | — | 20 | Desmethyl metabolite predominant; active | 7–20 | 80–100 |
| Amoxapine | — | — | — | 9-Hydroxy; 3–10 times as abundant; active | — | 200–400 |
| Maprotiline | 66–75 | 88 | 21–40 | Desmethylated, active | 52 | 200–300 |
| Trazodone | — | 73 | 8 | $m$-Chlorophenyl-piperazine; active | — | — |
| Fluoxetine | ? 72 | 94 | 24–96 | Norfluoxetine active | 20–45 | None found |
| Buproprion | — | 85 | 11–14 | ? Active | — | 25–100 |

the problem. Simple techniques such as fluid restriction, awakening the child to empty the bladder, use of simpler anticholinergic drugs, rewards for dry beds, and even alarm systems that go off when the bed is wet should be tried first (Kass et al., 1979). The beneficial effect of drug treatment lasts only for as long as the drug is given (see also Chapter 7).

## Chronic Pain

Clinicians in pain clinics have found tricyclics to be especially useful for treating a variety of chronically painful states that often cannot be definitely diagnosed. Whether such painful states represent depressive equivalents or whether such patients become secondarily depressed after some initial pain-producing insult is not clear. It is even possible that the tricyclics (sometimes phenothiazines are also used in combination) work directly on pain pathways. Generally doses used for treating chronic pain are similar to those used for treating depression (Stimmel and Escobar, 1986).

## Other Indications

Less frequent and less well-documented indications include the use of these drugs for treating obsessive-compulsive-phobic states, for treating children with school phobia, for treating children with minimal brain damage and hyperkinesis, for treating the attacks of cataplexy associated with narcolepsy, and for treating acute panic attacks.

# Efficacy

An extensive experience of more than 30 years of clinical use of antidepressants supports the contention that these are effective therapy. The extent to which antidepressants relieve depression has been more questionable. Only 60 to 70 percent of patients treated with these drugs attain any benefit, and many do not obtain complete remission. It is common for patients who have been severely acutely depressed to become chronically mildly depressed. This situation has been called "double depression," assuming the severe depression is a separate entity from the chronic depression, or dysthymia, as it has been called.

A survey of opinions about the type of response one might attain from tricyclic antidepressants indicated that the best response was seen in patients with primary (endogenous) depression with symptoms of early morning awakening, motor retardation, loss of appetite, weight loss, loss of interest in sex, loss of interest in work or hobbies, improved mood in the evening, and a prior response to tricyclic antidepressants. Amitriptyline was preferred for agitated depressions and imipramine for retarded depressions (Goldberg et al., 1988). It is difficult to determine how much such opinions are based on stereotypes and how much they are based on actual experience. For instance, no study has ever examined the question of the presumed selective responses to amitriptyline and imipramine. In any case, the general feeling is that endogenous depressions respond more specifically to tricyclics than do other types of depressions.

MAO inhibitors have been generally as effective for treating endogenous depressions as tricyclics. However, they are not as often used because of the problems associated with potential interactions with food or other drugs. Although their combination with tricyclics has been touted as being more effective than the latter drugs alone, at least two controlled comparisons have found that such combinations are no better than their individual components. Unfortunately, all these studies lacked statistical power to reject the null hypothesis (Pare, 1985).

Second-generation antidepressants are generally thought to be as effective as tricyclics, although such conclusions have been based on a relatively small number of controlled comparisons. Two of the newer drugs, trazodone and fluoxetine, may have advantages over the older ones in regard to side effects and dangers of overdose. The main advantage of having these additional drugs is that they afford alternative choices for patients who fail to respond to one of the older drugs.

Sympathomimetic stimulants have only limited effectiveness in special situations. Such conditions are more likely to be found by practicing psychiatrists dealing with individual patients than by clinical researchers. Relatively few studies have been done with these drugs, so experimental evidence regarding special areas of utility is scant.

Just as a number of controlled comparisons of ECT have shown it to be generally more effective than antidepressant drugs, so has a retrospective study. Patients who received ECT treatment for depression during the period 1959–1969 had marked or total improvement in 49 percent of cases, compared with a group that received antidepressant drugs, which had a rate of 27 percent such improvement (Avery and Winokur, 1977). The possibility remains that many of the patients treated with antidepressants were treated inadequately, but nonetheless, the study indicates the high reliability of ECT for treating depression.

# Choice of Drug

A complete history should include questions about previous responses to drug treatment. Lacking such information on the patient, the clinician should inquire about family members who may have been treated for depression, the assumption being that the etiologic type of depression may run true in close family members.

## Tricyclics

The choice of which tricyclic antidepressant to use in a particular patient is entirely empiric. Amitriptyline, which has the most effect on serotonin uptake and causes most sedation, has been contrasted with desipramine, which is a specific uptake inhibitor for norepinephrine with the least sedative effects. It has been averred that patients who do not respond to one should be tried on the other. No experimental evidence supports such a procedure. Indeed, it seems as though most patients, if they fail to respond to one tricyclic, will fail to respond to others, although exceptions occur. Despite all the new drugs that have become available, tricyclics must still be considered as the first-choice antidepressants.

## MAO Inhibitors

When it is evident that patients have responded to MAO inhibitors previously, or when patients suffer "atypical depressions," MAO inhibitors may be drugs of first choice. For other patients it is more or less a toss-up whether to try MAO inhibitors or second-generation drugs after the patient has failed with a tricyclic. If the choice is to try the MAO inhibitor, one need not wait for 2 weeks between treatment phases; the MAO inhibitor can be phased in as the tricyclic is phased out. Serious interactions from the combination have almost universally occurred following the opposite sequence of treatment.

## Second-Generation Drugs

Amoxapine and maprotiline offer no conspicuous advantages over tricyclic antidepressants. Whether patients who fail to respond to the latter drugs will respond to any of the second-generation drugs has not been adequately studied. If one is to try drugs of this class, trazodone and fluoxetine would be first choices.

## Sympathomimetics

Dextroamphetamine and methylphenidate have been used early in treatment with tricyclics, both to predict the ultimate response to the latter drugs as well as to help lift mood more quickly. They may also be useful in elderly patients, who often do not tolerate other types of antidepressants.

# Doses

The usual range of daily doses of antidepressants is shown in Table 4-3. At best, such ranges are only a rough guide. Clinical experience has shown that patients have responded to doses as low as 25 mg/day of tricyclics or that others may require doses of 600 mg/day for an adequate response. Such a wide dosage range tends to confirm the observation made many years ago that the range of plasma concentrations from the same dose of tricyclics may vary 30-fold. As the relationship between dose and plasma concentration is not predictable in individual patients, many clinicians feel that monitoring of plasma concentrations of those antidepressants for which a reasonable therapeutic range has been established may be more pertinent than relying solely on doses.

Most patients will attain plasma concentrations of a tricyclic antidepressant within the presumed therapeutic range on daily doses of 150 mg. In the absence of measurement of plasma concentrations, the presence of side effects should be a reasonable guide to dose. The usual practice is to push the dose until side

**Table 4-3.** Various Types of Antidepressant Drugs and Their Usual Daily Doses

| Drug | Dose (mg) |
|---|---|
| **Tricyclics** | |
| Imipramine | 75–200 |
| Desipramine | 75–200 |
| Amitriptyline | 75–200 |
| Nortriptyline | 75–150 |
| Protriptyline | 20–40 |
| Doxepin | 75–300 |
| Trimipramine | 75–200 |
| Clomipramine | 75–300 |
| **Monoamine Oxidase Inhibitors** | |
| Phenelzine | 45–75 |
| Tranylcypromine | 10–30 |
| Isocarboxazide | 20–50 |
| **Second-Generation** | |
| Amoxapine | 150–300 |
| Maprotiline | 75–300 |
| Trazodone | 50–600 |
| Fluoxetine | 20–60 |

effects become intolerable or the patient shows some clinical response. The absence of side effects, along with a failure to respond, is generally construed as evidence of inadequate plasma concentrations regardless of the dose of drug given.

Whenever doses are raised beyond the usual limits, it is well to monitor plasma concentrations, as some evidence suggests nonlinear kinetics with doses above 300 mg/day. The reasons for using such large doses should be well documented in the patients' records, as part of the current practice of defensive medicine.

## Dosage Schedules

The usual dosage schedule for initiating treatment with tricyclic antidepressants has been to use divided daily doses, such as 25 mg three times daily, and then to increase by increments of 25 to 50 mg/day to the desired therapeutic dose. Such schedules almost mandate that steady-state concentrations of effective plasma levels will not be reached until more than a week of treatment has passed. Thus, the delay in response to these drugs could be more likely a pharmacokinetic than a pharmacodynamic phenomenon. Once a therapeutic dose range has been reached, it is possible to consolidate doses so that a single dose, usually given at night, can be given. With MAO inhibitors it is possible to give the full therapeutic dose from the very beginning (usually 1 mg/kg/day of phenelzine). With drugs that tend to stimulate patients, such as sympathomimetics or fluoxetine, giving doses earlier in the day is more reasonable.

If situations can be contrived at home to mimic those that prevail in hospital, initial full oral doses of tricyclics may be given. When the drug is administered in this fashion, response is often much faster than following conventional dosage schedules. A more rapid onset of action has also been reported from parenteral doses of tricyclics, either by slow intravenous drip or intramuscular administration.

## Pattern of Clinical Response

Because of the slow rate of recovery, some patients may become discouraged with treatment and terminate it prematurely. Patience should be counseled. Sleep disorder may be the first symptom to be alleviated, with mood elevation taking more time. Responses of patients have varied considerably, some responding within a few days and others not responding for 6 or even 12 weeks. The contention has been made that early responses represent nonspecific responses (patients would have gone into remission anyway) whereas true drug responses take a much longer period of time (Quitkin et al., 1987). Such logic defies an old clinical axiom that the longer it takes for a patient to respond to a treatment the more likely the response is nonspecific. One should always be leery of dramatic responses, which may signify that the patient has found the solution to existing problems by ending their existence.

## Refractory Patients

Almost one-third of patients treated with antidepressants fail to respond to the first trial of treatment. Definitions of treatment-resistance vary, but one might argue that failure to respond, even though less than optimally, after 3 to 4 weeks of treatment is cause for concern. Should the patient actually get worse or entertain suicidal thoughts, the situation borders on the critical. A reasonable approach to these problems is to consider the four Ds: diagnosis, dose and duration of treatment, drug, or a different treatment.

Diagnosis must be re-examined constantly. Could the patient's depression be secondary to another drug being used for medical treatment? Many are possible (Hollister, 1986). Could it be secondary to some medical problem, such as an occult malignancy? Is the patient in a depressive phase of manic-depressive disorder, in which case lithium might be indicated? Is the patient suffering from a delusional or agitated depression, or a schizoaffective disorder, each of which may respond to the addition of an antipsychotic? Or is the patient in the early stage of progressive dementia, which might be made worse by the anticholinergic effects of tricyclics?

Has enough dose been given of the current drug to assure a therapeutic plasma concentration? Patients who fail to respond to a tricyclic but who have few side effects should be treated with doses of at least 300 mg/day with determination of plasma concentrations before assuming that the drug has failed (Wager and Klein, 1988). The primary indication for a measurement of plasma concentrations of an antidepressant is failure to respond to usual therapeutic doses. Low concentrations may reflect a bioavailability problem or noncompliance, each of which must be dealt with separately. Moderate concentrations may not be adequate for a particular patient; the dose may have to be increased further. If concentrations are considerably above the usual therapeutic range, a trial with lowered doses (especially in the case of nortriptyline) might be worth trying. The proper length of treatment is controversial. One should attempt to alleviate depression as rapidly as possible, bearing in mind both the consequences or prolonged morbidity as well as the personal suffering of the depressed patient. The illness also has an appreciable mortality rate that prompt treatment might mitigate.

Whether to try next another tricyclic or switch to another class of antidepressant drug is a matter of clinical judgment. Often patients who have failed to respond to a tricyclic may respond to a MAO inhibitor. Even those patients who do not respond to conventional doses of an MAO inhibitor may require unusually large doses, such as 120 to 200 mg/day of tranylcypromine, before responding (Guze et al., 1987). One of the newer antidepressants should probably be tried after the older drugs have failed.

Many different adjunctive treatments have been recommended for managing treatment-resistant patients. The addition of lithium is best documented, presumably based on an action of lithium on serotonergic systems (De Montigny et al., 1983). Other treatments that are either still experimental or controversial include addition of thyroid hormone in euthyroid patients; combination of a tricyclic with an MAO inhibitor; dextroamphetamine or methylphenidate added to tricyclics; neurotransmitter precursors, such as tryptophan; and manipulations of the sleep–wake cycle. Experience with the addition of thyroid hormones has been substantial. Nine of 12 patients refractory to tricyclics alone showed improvement after the addition of 25 to 50 $\mu$g/day doses of liothyronine ($T_3$). Just why such small doses of thyroid hormone in presumably euthyroid patients alleviate depression is still unclear (Goodwin et al., 1982). Which of these various adjunctive treatments to try first is a matter of clinical judgment.

The most effective adjunctive treatment by far is electroconvulsive therapy (ECT). ECT can generally be used in conjunction with most prevailing drug treatments. Fewer treatments might be needed and remissions might last longer if ECT is combined with drug therapy.

## Continuation and Maintenance Treatment

One assumes that each depressive episode has a finite duration. The problem is that one cannot be sure at what point in its course the patient was first seen or how long the course will be in a particular patient. Thus, treatment must be continued beyond the point of remission to prevent early relapse. Such continuation treatment is measured in weeks or months. Another aspect of depressive illness is that episodes tend to recur. In patients who already have had at least one recurrence of depression, it is reasonable to assume that maintenance treatment might prevent others. Such treatment is measured in years.

The duration of continuation treatment was explored in a collaborative project. Withdrawal of antidepressant treatment was safe only after the patient had been free of symptoms for 16 to 20 weeks. Mild as well as severe symptoms need to be considered in making the decision (Prien and Kupfer, 1986). Whether such continuation treatment requires full therapeutic doses of antidepressants or can be accomplished with lesser doses has not been examined.

The risk of relapse into an episode of depression was examined in 141 patients followed for a median period of 62 weeks. Older age of onset as well as having had three or more prior episodes of depression predicted a significantly greater likelihood of relapse (Keller et al., 1983). Thus, the natural history of the disorder in individual patients must be considered in making decisions about maintenance therapy.

Maintenance therapy with imipramine, lithium, and a combination of the two drugs was examined in patients with both unipolar and bipolar affective disorders. Lithium, as well as the combination, was superior for preventing relapses of bipolar affective episodes. The combination was no better than lithium alone, suggesting that the latter drug was most important. On the other hand, imipramine and the combination were superior in preventing relapses in unipolar depressions, with the combination being no better (Prien et al., 1984). Thus, the notion of using lithium to prevent relapse in bipolar illness and tricyclics for prevention of relapse in unipolar depressions was confirmed.

## Depression in the Elderly

Depression is common in elderly patients (Blazer, 1989). Pervasive depression in the elderly has been characterized as having at least one of the following symptoms: depression lasting at least one day or longer; depression that is not easily shaken off; crying; bleak outlook toward the future; and at least one of the following symptoms or signs: worrying disproportionate to cause that cannot be controlled; looks depressed throughout interview. Using such a definition, 13 percent of an elderly sample of subjects in New York were judged to be depressed as compared with 10 percent in London (Gurland et al., 1985). Loss, a key concept in the psychology of depression, is frequent in older patients: loss of vigor, companionship, social position, income, as well as the cumulative losses of a lifetime. Whether aging creates a biologic predisposition to depression through changes in catecholamines is only speculative.

Depression in the elderly patient can be accompanied by unusual symptoms such as social withdrawal and confusion (which might be construed as signs of dementia) or delusions of persecution and hostile behavior (which might be construed as evidence of psychosis) or chronic hypochondriasis (which might lead to detailed and fruitless medical investigations). In addition, many of the drugs that elderly patients take for medical purposes may cause depression, or many of the illnesses they suffer may produce a secondary depression (Goff and Jenike, 1986). Thus, making a secure diagnosis may be difficult, and more options for treatment must be considered.

When a decision has been made to use antidepressant drugs, one must choose from the existing array, but choose carefully. Most tricyclics have anticholinergic and sedative side effects that may be poorly tolerated; desipramine seems to have the least. Imipramine is reputed to be more likely than others to produce orthostatic hypotension. MAO inhibitors, which are often useful in elderly depressed, also produce orthostatic hypotension. The presence of cardiac disease in itself is not a contraindication to use of tricyclics, but a relative contraindication exists in the presence of atrioventricular or intraventricular heart block. Whether or not newer drugs, such as trazodone, fluoxetine, and buproprion, may be preferable to the older drugs remains to be proved.

Opinion is somewhat divided regarding doses of drugs to be used in elderly patients. Some investigators believe that full doses, comparable to what are used in younger patients, are required to produce therapeutic plasma concentrations; others are convinced that doses should be much more conservative. Thus, the range of tricyclic daily doses may be 25 to 75 mg in elderly patients and still produce not only therapeutic plasma concentrations but also a desired clinical response (Salzman, 1985).

Because of the many psychological factors that may make elderly patients depressed, various psychotherapies should be strongly considered. Cognitive, behavioral, and social approaches have been used successfully in both nonendogenous and endogenous depressions in the elderly (Gallagher and Thompson, 1983). However, the more endogenous the depression and the more severe its manifestations, the more likely it is that drug therapy will be required.

## Monitoring Plasma Concentrations

Whether routine monitoring of plasma concentrations is a cost-effective procedure remains controversial. Proponents maintain that early adjustment of doses to attain a plasma concentration in the presumed therapeutic range will shorten the time to response and reduce total days in hospital. Those who doubt routine monitoring point out that therapeutic ranges (summarized in Table 4-2) vary widely, that they have not been established for many drugs, and that for almost every report defining such a range, another has failed. A blind controlled trial of the value of routine monitoring with feedback of the information to the treating physician resulted in neither more time spent within the presumed therapeutic range for nortriptyline nor a more favorable outcome than among patients similarly monitored but without such information being available (Hollister et al., 1980).

Blood for plasma concentrations should be obtained in the postabsorptive state, about 10 to 12 hours after the last dose. Even when sampling time is constant, the same patient may show a fair degree of variation in both the total plasma concentration and the division of parent drug and metabolites while on a constant dose at steady-state conditions.

What might be the indications for ordering a determination of plasma concentration of tricyclics? The following are some possibilities:

1. A patient has received a presumably adequate dose but has failed to

respond. The finding of a plasma concentration markedly below the therapeutic range would be an indication that something is amiss. On the other hand, if the plasma concentration is in the therapeutic range, but not excessively high, one might feel encouraged to increase the dose as long as clinical toxicity was not evident.

2. If a patient has a side effect that is uncertainly related to drug therapy, the presence of very high plasma concentrations might resolve the issue.
3. Whenever one feels constrained to use higher than usual doses of these drugs, monitoring plasma concentrations might help avoid problems and would demonstrate a degree of prudence. Doses of 300 mg or more of amitriptyline or imipramine tend to produce very high plasma concentrations. One should limit levels to less than 600 ng/ml of combined drug and metabolite. No current evidence supports increasing plasma concentrations further.
4. When treating very old or very young patients, one might wish to check plasma concentrations to keep them low.
5. The presence of intercurrent illness may be a reason to lower plasma concentrations to the lower limits of potential therapeutic efficacy. Illness may decrease the degree of protein binding of drugs, decrease their metabolism, or increase the susceptibility of the patient to adverse effects of the drug.
6. In cases of drug overdose, plasma concentrations may be particularly useful late in the course when making a decision about when to relax vigilance. A plasma concentration that has returned to the therapeutic range, as well as clinical evidence of remission, would make one feel secure removing the patient from intensive care. Such determinations would not be especially useful early in the course of intoxication, for the level of drug has relatively little bearing on the subsequent clinical course of the intoxication; that is best judged by the prevailing clinical appearance of the patient.

## Combinations

The combination of a tricyclic antidepressant with an MAO inhibitor must still be regarded as experimental. Combining two antidepressants, whether tricyclics or others, has no substantive support. Sympathomimetic stimulants may be combined with tricyclics with possible benefit. Combinations with antipsychotic drugs are commonly employed and may be helpful; such combinations are best made extemporaneously. Concurrent use of antidepressants and benzodiazepines is safe, but whether such combinations have any specific advantage is difficult to tell. Many of the adjunctive treatments already mentioned for managing resistant patients have been safely combined with antidepressants. Serotonin precursors, such as l-tryptophan, should not be combined with serotonin uptake inhibitors, such as fluoxetine. MAO inhibitors should also be avoided in patients treated with fluoxetine.

## Age Limitations

Tricyclics should be used cautiously in children or in adults past age 50. Protein-binding may be decreased in either extreme of life, but increased unbound drug may be less important in contributing to exaggerated drug effects than impaired metabolism in the elderly. Whether or not the elderly are overly sensitive to pharmacodynamic actions of these drugs is difficult to show, but clinical experience suggests that they are.

## Suicidal Risks

Suicide is most likely to occur in patients with severe depressions, in those with a family history of suicide, or in those who have made previous attempts. Concurrent physical illness, alcoholism, or estrangement from family also increase the risk. A patient who during treatment shows an abrupt change for no apparent reason is at risk. Sudden improvement may simply signify that the patient has decided on suicide as the solution for his problems. Sudden rejection of help may signify a feeling of hopelessness that may be resolved by suicide. Psychiatric referral and hospitalization are indicated whenever suicide is considered to be a risk, although obviously in some cases nothing prevents this outcome.

## Adverse Effects

Adverse effects of antidepressants are summarized in Table 4-4. Most common unwanted effects are minor, but they may seriously affect the acceptability of drug treatment by the patient; the more seriously depressed the patient is, the better unwanted effects are tolerated. Most normal persons find all but the smallest doses of these drugs somewhat disagreeable (Blackwell, 1985).

### Sedative Effects

These effects are generally dose related. They are highly variable with trazodone and least likely to occur with protriptyline, fluoxetine, and buproprion.

### Sympathomimetic Actions

These effects of various antidepressants may be obscured by other more prominent actions on the autonomic nervous system, but they are explainable on the basis of known pharmacologic actions of most of these drugs. Tremor is extremely common; treatment with a beta-blocking drug, such as propranolol, may be helpful.

### Anticholinergic Activity

Treatment with a peripherally acting cholinomimetic, bethanechol, may counter the peripheral anticholinergic action of the tricyclics. Precipitation of

**Table 4-4.** Side Effects of Antidepressants

| Side Effect | Occurrence |
|---|---|
| Sedation | |
| Lassitude, fatigue, sleepiness | Assume that all antidepressants may |
| Impaired function with alcohol and other drugs | produce these effects; fluoxetine and buproprion probably less likely |
| Sympathomimetic | |
| Tachycardia, tremor, sweating | All tricyclics |
| Insomnia | Fluoxetine most likely |
| Agitation, aggravation of psychosis | All |
| Anticholinergic | |
| Blurred vision, aggravation of glaucoma | All tricyclics, less likely with fluoxetine, trazodone, buproprion |
| Constipation | |
| Urinary hesitancy | |
| Fuzzy thinking, delirium | |
| Neurologic | |
| Paresthesias, neuropathy | All tricyclics |
| EEG abnormalities, seizures | Maprotiline, buproprion more likely |
| Psychiatric | |
| Confusion, central anticholinergic syndrome, withdrawal | All tricyclics |
| Cardiovascular | |
| Orthostatic hypotension | All tricyclics |
| Delayed cardiac conduction | All tricyclics, dose-related |
| Arrhythmias, sudden death | Uncertain |
| Allergic/Toxic | |
| Cholestatic jaundice | Rare with all |
| Agranulocytosis | |
| Metabolic/Endocrine | |
| Weight gain | Tricyclics |
| Sexual disturbances | Variable; priapism with trazodone |
| Dysmorphogenesis | Uncertain |

narrow-angle glaucoma seems to be mentioned more frequently than it actually occurs. It appears that some of the second-generation compounds are less likely to produce anticholinergic effects than older drugs.

## Cardiovascular Effects

Palpitation, tachycardia, and orthostatic hypotension were recognized early as unwanted effects of these drugs. Later, arrhythmia and electrocardiographic abnormalities were described. More serious cardiovascular side effects have generally been associated with overdoses. Prolonged atrioventricular or intraventricular conduction is a relative contraindication to tricyclics. Some second-generation drugs may be preferable for patients with heart disease.

## Psychiatric Reactions

Confusional reactions are most often seen in patients over the age of 40 years treated with tricyclics. The situation may be made worse if the patient is also receiving other drugs with anticholinergic action, such as antipsychotics or antiparkinson drugs.

A central anticholinergic syndrome consisting of delirium, anxiety, hyperactivity, hallucinations, disorientation, and seizures has been described for many drugs with anticholinergic action, especially when taken in combination. A good general rule is that any patient showing new or bizarre mental symptoms while on antidepressants should have the drug discontinued until the situation can be appraised. Some patients may become agitated and manic with tricyclics, but one should always consider the possibility that, rather than this representing a drug effect, they are really manic-depressive.

Withdrawal reactions have been described as a rare complication of terminating tricyclic administration. Motor restlessness and cholinergic symptoms and signs predominate, but such reactions are seldom serious. Occasionally, these symptoms may be mistaken for depressive relapse.

## Neurologic Effects

Paresthesias may herald the rare development of peripheral neuropathy. Seizures are rare with most antidepressants except maprotiline and buproprion; they are dose related.

## Allergic or Toxic Reactions

Rashes are uncommon. Cholestatic jaundice and agranulocytosis have been reported in the past but are now so rare as to hardly merit consideration.

## Metabolic and Endocrine Effects

Weight gain is frequent with tricyclics, just as it is with the phenothiazines. Part of the gain may be due to increased appetite with remission of depression, but part is probably due to a central action.

The syndrome of inappropriate secretion of antidiuretic hormone has been reported from time to time with various tricyclics.

## Dysmorphogenesis

This issue, as with so many drugs, remains open. Evidence that these drugs have such effects is not very persuasive. One must accept the conventional wisdom that unless a drug is necessary for preserving life or maintaining adequate function, it should not be used in pregnancy.

# Drug Interactions

## Pharmacodynamic

Many of these interactions have already been discussed. Sedative effects may be additive with other sedatives, especially with alcoholic beverages. Patients placed on tricyclics should be warned that use of alcohol may lead to greater than usual impairment of driving ability.

Thioridazine is often used to treat depressed patients, sometimes in combination with tricyclic antidepressants. Because thioridazine has the same anti-arrhythmic and atropine-line effects on the heart as do the tricyclics, the possibility of adverse cardiac effect may be increased by such a combination.

The anticholinergic action of tricyclics may be additive with that of anti-psychotic or antiparkinson drugs. The latter are generally unnecessary when tricyclics are combined with antipsychotics. Mental confusion may be the predominant symptom of the excessive anticholinergic activity.

Reversal of the antihypertensive action of guanethidine is a most dramatic interaction. The blood pressure not only quickly returns to elevated levels, but may "overshoot" to dangerous levels. Guanethidine is concentrated in sympathetic nerve endings by the same amine pump blocked by tricyclics. Thus, it is prevented from reaching its site of action. A similar reversal of action of other antihypertensives, such as methyldopa and clonidine, has been described (Ka Kit Hui, 1983).

The many interactions of MAO inhibitors with foods (cheeses, yeast extracts, certain alcoholic beverages, and other foods) are well known. Current thinking is that overconcern about such interactions has diminished the utility of these drugs (Folks, 1983). Patients should be warned about the possibility of acute hypertensive reactions from interactions of MAO inhibitors and various foods or other drugs.

## Pharmacokinetic

Various pharmacokinetic interactions between tricyclics and other drugs continue to be reported, but their clinical significance is questionable. Not only is there a pharmacodynamic interaction between ethanol and amitriptyline, but ethanol in close proximity to a dose of amitriptyline markedly increased the amount of unbound drug in blood as well as decreasing its clearance (Dorian et al., 1983). Whether such conditions prevail during chronic therapy has not been investigated. Thioridazine inhibits the metabolism of desipramine, leading to higher concentrations of the latter drug (Hirschowitz et al., 1983). Such a combination is best avoided for reasons mentioned earlier.

Cimetidine, because of its ability to inhibit both demethylation and hydroxlation as well as to reduce hepatic clearance of drugs, might be expected to interact with tricyclics. As expected, the bioavailability of imipramine was increased but not that of nortriptyline; the bioavailability of 10-hydroxy-nortriptyline was also increased. Results were highly variable between subjects, making generalization difficult (Henauer and Hollister, 1984).

# OVERDOSES
## Tricyclics

Tricyclics are extremely dangerous drugs when taken in overdose. Depressed patients are more likely to be suicidal than other patients. Thus, we have a paradox in which patients at high risk are given drugs with a high risk. Prescriptions should be limited to amounts less than 1.25 g, or 50 dose units of 25 mg. If one suspects the possible use of these drugs for suicidal purposes, their care should be entrusted to a family member. At all costs, they should be kept away from children.

Both accidental and deliberate overdoses of these drugs are frequent; they are a serious medical emergency. Major symptoms include: (1) coma with shock and sometimes metabolic acidosis; (2) respiratory depression with a tendency to sudden apnea; (3) agitation or delirium both before and after consciousness is obtunded; (4) neuromuscular irritability and seizures; (5) hyperpyrexia; (6) bowel and bladder paralysis; and (7) a great variety of cardiac manifestations, including conduction defects and arrhythmias. Cardiac problems are the principal distinguishing features.

Management of cardiac problems is difficult. Antiarrhythmic drugs having the least effect on decreasing cardiac conduction should be used. Lidocaine, propranolol, and phenytoin have been used successfully, but quinidine and procainamide are contraindicated. Continual cardiac monitoring is essential, with provisions at hand for resuscitation. Arterial blood gasses and pH should be measured frequently, as both hypoxia and metabolic acidosis predispose to arrhythmias. Sodium bicarbonate and intravenous potassium chloride may be required to restore acid–base balance or to correct hypokalemia; such measures may adequately manage arrhythmias. Electrical pacing must be used in refractory cases.

Other treatment is entirely supportive. After placement of a cuffed endotracheal tube, attempts should be made to remove residual drug from the gastrointestinal tract. Absorption may be slow due to the strong anticholinergic effects. Activated charcoal may bind the drug and then allow for further removal by catharsis. Ventilatory assistance is of prime importance. Shock is best treated with fluids or plasma expanders. Hyperpyrexia is treated by cooling. Seizures may be treated with intravenous phenytoin (which may also double as an antiarrhythmic agent) or diazepam. Patients should not be discharged until they have been conscious for a day or two and most abnormal signs have disappeared. Measurement of plasma concentrations of the drug may be helpful in making the decision about the safety of discharge. Virtually all recovered patients have avoided any permanent residual effects.

## Monoamine Oxidase Inhibitors

Intoxication with MAO inhibitors is unusual. Agitation, delirium, and neuromuscular excitability are followed by obtunded consciousness, seizures, shock, and hyperthermia. Supportive treatment is generally adequate, although sedatives with alpha-adrenergic receptor blocking action, such as chlorpromazine, may be useful.

## Second-Generation Compounds

Amoxapine lacks cardiotoxicity as compared with tricyclics, but has significantly more neurotoxicity. Coma, seizures, and, less frequently, renal failure have followed overdoses. Seizures may be extremely difficult to control. Maprotiline is similar in toxicity to tricyclics, but causing seizures more frequently (Crome and Ali, 1986). Overdoses of trazodone have been marked by extreme sedation but generally have not required much treatment; although instances of ventricular tachycardia have been reported on therapeutic doses, such occurrences have been notably absent in overdoses. Overdoses of fluoxetine have only rarely been fatal. Two deaths occurred among nearly 40 instances, but other drugs were also present. Nausea, vomiting, and CNS excitation have been prominent symptoms. Overdoses up to 1400 mg have been survived without incident (Finnegan and Gabiola, 1988). Thus, some second-generation drugs seem to have realized the promise of less difficulty from overdoses.

## REFERENCES

Aronson MD, Hafez H (1986) A case of trazodone-induced ventricular tachycardia. J Clin Psychiatry 48:388–389

Avery D, Winokur G (1977) The efficacy of electroconvulsive therapy and antidepressants in depression. Biol Psychiatry 12:506–523

Barbaccia ML, Ravizza L, Costa E (1986) Maprotiline: an antidepressant with an unusual pharmacological profile. J Pharmacol Exp Ther 236:307–312

Benedetti MS, Dostert P (1985) Sterochemical aspects of MAO interactions: reversible and selective inhibitors of monoamine oxidase. Trends Pharmacol Sci 246–251

Benfield P, Ward A (1986) Fluvoxamine. A review of its pharmacodynamic and pharmacokinetic properties, and therapeutic efficacy in depressive illness. Drugs 32:313–334

Blackwell B (1985) pp 24–61. In Dukes MNG (ed): Meyler's Side Effects of Drugs. Elsevier, Amsterdam

Blazer A (1989) Depression in the elderly. N Engl J Med 320:164–166

Bowden CL, Koslow SH, Hanin I, et al (1985) Effects of amitriptyline and imipramine on brain amine neurotransmitter metabolites in cerebrospinal fluid. Clin Pharmacol Ther 37:316–324

Burch JE, Ahmed O, Hullin RP, Mindham RHS (1988) Antidepressive effect of amitriptyline treatment with drug levels controlled within three different ranges. Psychopharmacology 94:197–205

Butler AD (1986) Letter. My dear colleague: Are you considering suicide? JAMA 255:2599–2600

Byerley WF, McConnell EJ, McCabe RT, et al (1988) Decreased beta-adrenergic receptors in rat brain after chronic administration of the selective serotonin uptake inhibitor, fluoxetine. Psychopharmacology 94:141–143

Coccaro EF, Siever LJ (1985) Second generation antidepressants: a comparative review. J Clin Psychopharmacol 25:241–260

Cooper BR, Hester TJ, Maxwell RA (1980) Behavioral and biochemical effects of the antidepressant buproprion (Wellbutrin): evidence for selective blockade of dopamine uptake in vivo. J Pharmacol Exp Ther 215:127–134

Crome P, Ali C (1986) Clinical features and management of self-poisoning with newer antidepressants. Med Toxicol 1:411–420

Davidson J, McLeod MN, White HL (1978) Inhibition of platelet monoamine oxidase in depression subjects treated with phenelzine. Am J Psychiatry 135:470–472

Davidson JRT, Giller EL, Zisook S, Overall JE (1988) An efficacy study of isocarboxazid and placebo in depression, and its relationship to depressive nosology. Arch Gen Psychiatry 45:120–127

Davis KL, Hollister LE, Mathe AA, et al (1981) Neuroendocrine and neurochemical measurements in depression. Am J Psychiatry 138:1555–1562

De Montigny C, Cournoyer G, Morissette R, et al (1983) Lithium carbonate addition in tricyclic antidepressant-resistant unipolar depression. Arch Gen Psychiatry 40:1327–1334

De Montigny C, Grunberg F, Mayer A, Deschens JP (1981) Lithium induces rapid relief of depression in tricyclic antidepressant non-responders. Br J Psychiatry 138:252–256

Dessain EC, Schatzberg AF, Woods BT, Cole JE (1986) Maprotiline treatment of depression. A perspective on seizures. Arch Gen Psychiatry 43:86–90

Dorian P, Sellers EM, Reed KL (1983) Amitriptyline and ethanol: pharmacokinetic and pharmacodynamic interaction. Eur J Clin Pharmacol 25:325–331

Feighner JP, Aden GC, Fabre LF, et al (1983) Comparison of alprazolam, imipramine and placebo in the treatment of depression. JAMA 249:3057–3064

Feighner JP, Boyer WR (1988) Overview of controlled trials of trazodone in clinical expression. Psychopharmacology 95:S50–S53

Finnegan K, Gabiola J (1988) Fluoxetine overdose. Am J Psychiatry 145:1604

Folks DG (1983) Monoamine oxidase inhibitors: reappraisal of dietary considerations. J Clin Psychopharmacol 3:249–252

Gallagher DE, Thompson LW (1983) Effectiveness of psychotherapy for both endogenous and nonendogenous depression in older adult outpatients. J Gerontol 38:707–720

Goff DC, Jenike MA (1986) Treatment-resistant depression in the elderly. J Am Geriatr Soc 34:63–70

Goldberg SC, Tilley DH, Friedel RO, et al (1988) Who benefits from tricyclic antidepressants: a survey. J Clin Psychiatry 49:224–228

Goodwin FK, Prange A, Post R, et al (1982) Potentiation of antidepressant effects by 1-triiodothyronine in tricyclic non-responders. Am J Psychiatry 139:34–38

Green AR (1987) Evolving concepts on the interactions between antidepressant treatments and monoamine neurotransmitters. Neuropharmacology 26:815–822

Gurland BJ, Wilder DE, Copeland J (1985) Concepts of depression in the elderly: signposts to future mental health needs, pp 443–451. In Gaitz CM, Samorajski T (eds): Aginign 2000: Our Health Care Destiny. Springer-Verlag, New York

Guze BH, Baxter LR Jr, Rego J (1987) Refractory depression treated with high doses of monoamine oxidase inhibitor. J Clin Psychiatry 48:31–32

Henauer SA, Hollister LE (1984) Cimetidine interaction with imipramine and nortriptyline. Clin Pharmacol Ther 35:183–187

Hirschowitz J, Bennett JA, Zemlan FP, Garver DL (1983) Thioridazine effect on desipramine plasma levels. J Clin Psychopharmacol 3:376–379

Hollister LE (1986) Drug-induced psychiatric disorders and their management. Med Toxicol 1:428–448

Hollister LE, Davis KL, Overall JE, Anderson T (1978) Excretion of MHPG in normal subjects. Implications for biological classification of affective disorders. Arch Gen Psychiatry 35:1410–1415

Hollister LE, Overall JE, Pokorny A, Shelton J (1971) Acetophenazine and diazepam in anxious depressions. Arch Gen Psychiatry 24:273–278

Hollister LE, Pfefferbaum A, Davis KL (1980) Monitoring nortriptyline plasma concentrations. Am J Psychiatry 137:485–486

Jue SG, Dawson GW, Brogden RN (1982) Amoxapine: a review of its pharmacology and efficacy in depressed states. Drugs 24:1–23

Ka Kit Hui (1983) Hypertensive crisis induced by interaction of clonidine with imipramine. J Am Geriatr Ass 31:164–165

Kass EJ, Diokno AC, Montealegre A (1979) Enuresis: principles of management and result of treatment. J Urol 121:794–796

Keller MB, Lavori PW, Lewis CE, Klerman GL (1983) Predictors of relapse in major depressive disorder. JAMA 250:3299–3304

Kent TA, Preskorn SH, Glotzbach RK, Irwin GH (1986) Amitriptyline normalizes tetrabenazine-induced changes in cerebral microcirculation. Biol Psychiatry 21:483–491

Klein HE, Muller N (1985) Trazodone in endogenous depressed patients: a negative report and a critical evaluation of the pertaining literature. Prog Neuropsychopharmacol Biol Psychiatry 9:173–186

Kuhn R (1958) The treatment of depressive states with G22355 (imipramine hydrochloride). Am J Psychiatry 115:459

Mann JJ, Aarons SF, Wilner PJ, et al (1989) A controlled study of the antidepressant efficacy of (-)-deprenyl. A selective monoamine oxidase inhibitor. Arch Gen Psychiatry 46:45 50

Muscettola G, Potter WZ, Pickar D, Goodwin FK (1984) Urinary 3-methoxy-4-hydroxyphenylglycol and major affective disorders. A replication and new findings. Arch Gen Psychiatry 41:337–342

Myers JK, Weissman MM, Tischler GL, et al (1984) Six-month prevalence of psychiatric disorders in three communities. Arch Gen Psychiatry 41:959–967

Nierenberg AA, Feinstein AR (1988) How to evaluate a diagnostic test. Lessons from the rise and fall of dexamethasone suppression test. JAMA 259:1699–1702

Nordin C, Bertilsson L, Siwers B (1987) Clinical and biochemical effects during treatment of depression with nortriptyline: the role of 10-hydroxynortriptyline. Clin Pharmacol Ther 42:10–19

Pare CMP (1985) The present status of monoamine oxidase inhibitors. Br J Psychiatry 146:576–584

Pokorny A (1983) Prediction of suicide in psychiatric patients. Report of a prospective study. Arch Gen Psychiatry 40:249–257

Prien RF, Kupfer DJ (1986) Continuation drug therapy for major depressive episodes: how long should it be maintained? Am J Psychiatry 143:18–23

Prien RF, Kupfer DJ, Mansky PA, et al (1984) Drug therapy in the prevention of recurrences in unipolar and bipolar affective disorders. Report of the NIMH Collaborative Study Group comparing lithium carbonate, imipramine and a lithium carbonate–imipramine combination. Arch Gen Psychiatry 41:1096–1104

Quitkin FM, Rabkin JD, Markowitz JM, et al (1987) Use of pattern analysis to identify true drug response. A Replication. Arch Gen Psychiatry 44:259–264

Quitkin FM, Stewart JW, McGrath PJ, et al (1988) Phenelzine versus imipramine in the treatment of probably atypical depression: defining syndrome boundaries of selective MAOI responders. Am J Psychiatry 145:306–311

Rigal JG, Albin HC, Duchier AR, et al (1987) Imipramine blood levels and clinical outcome. J Clin Psychopharmacology 7:222–229

Robins LN, Helzer JE, Weissman MM, et al (1984) Lifetime prevalence of specific psychiatric disorders in three sites. Arch Gen Psychiatry 41:949–958

Robinson DS, Nies A, Ravaris CL, et al (1978) Clinical pharmacology of phenelzine. Arch Gen Psychiatry 35:629–635

Rudzik AD, Hester JB, Tang AH, et al (1973) Triazolobenzodiazepines, new class of central nervous system depressant compounds. pp 285–297. In Garattini S, Mussini E, Randall LO (eds): The Benzodiazepines. Raven Press, New York

Salzman C (1985) Clinical guidelines for the use of antidepressant drugs in geriatric patients. J Clin Psychiatry 46 (sec 2):38–44

Schatzberg AF, Dessain E, O'Neil P, et al (1987) Recent studies on selective serotonergic antidepressants: trazodone, fluoxetine and fluvoxamine. J Clin Psychopharmacology 7:44S–49S

Silvestrini B, Valeri P (1984) Trazodone, a new avenue in the treatment of depression. Psychopathology 17 (suppl 2):3–14

Sommi RW, Crismon ML, Bowden CL (1987) Fluoxetine: a serotonin-specific second-generation antidepressant. Pharmacotherapy 7:1–15

Soroko FE, Mehta NB, Maxwell RA, et al (1977) Buproprion hydrochloride. A novel antidepressant agent. J Pharm Pharmacol 29:767–770

Stahl SM, Palazidou L (1986) The pharmacology of depression: studies of neurotransmitter receptors lead the search for biochemical lesions and new drug therapies. Trends Pharmacol Sci 349–353

Stimmel GL, Escobar JI (1986) Antidepressants in chronic pain. Pharmacotherapy 6:262–267

Stokes PE, Stoll PM, Koslow SH, et al (1984) Pretreatment DST and hypothalamic-pituitary-adrenocortinal function in depressed patients and comparison groups. Arch Gen Psychiatry 41:257–267

Sulser F (1987) Serotonin-norepinephrine receptor interactions in the brain: implications for the pharmacology and pathophysiology of affective disorders. J Clin Psychiatry 48 (suppl):12–18

Sutfin TA, DeVane L, Jusko WJ (1984) The analysis and disposition of imipramine and its active metabolites in man. Psychopharmacology 82:310–317

Vallejo J, Castro C, Catalan R, Salamero M (1987) Double-blind study of imipramine versus phenelzine in melancholias and dysthymic disorders. Br J Psychiatry 151:639–642

Vetulani J, Sansone M, Baran L, Hano J (1984) Opposite action of *m*-chlorophenyl-piperazine on avoidance depression induced by trazodone and pimozide in CD-1 mice. Psychopharmacology 83:166–168

Vetulani J, Sulser F (1975) Action of various antidepressant treatments reduces reactivity of noradrenergic cyclic AMP-generating system in limbic forebrain. Nature (London) 495:495–496

Vogel GW (1983) Evidence for REM sleep deprivation as the mechanism of action of antidepressant drugs. Prog Neuropsychopharmacol Biol Psychiatry 7:343–349

Wager SG, Klein DF (1988) Drug therapy strategies for treatment-resistant depression. Psychopharmacol Bull 24:69–74

Warner MD, Peabody CA, Whiteford HA, Hollister LE (1987) Trazodone and priapism. J Clin Psychiatry 48:244–245

Zeller EA, ed (1959) Amine oxidase inhibitors. Ann NY Acad Sci 80:551–1045

# 5

---

# ANTIPSYCHOTIC DRUGS

## HISTORY

Antipsychotic drugs have been used clinically for almost 35 years. Their impact on psychiatry, specifically in the treatment of schizophrenia, has been great. First, they have markedly reduced the number of patients chronically hospitalized in mental institutions. Second, they have markedly shifted psychiatric thinking to a more biologic basis. Unfortunately, neither of these developments has been as rewarding as initially hoped. The tragedy of a fruitless life is now being played out in sleazy boarding houses or skid-row hotels rather than in mental institutions.

Most discouraging is that more effective pharmacotherapy has not been developed. Present drugs have many deficiencies: They are not curative; their ameliorative effects are often limited; many patients remain totally unresponsive; they are unpleasant to take, so that many patients are less than fully compliant; they produce major side effects, such as tardive dyskinesia, whose full implications are still uncertain.

Advances in drug design have resulted in the development of highly potent agents or depot preparations that permit better compliance or drugs with more specific actions on dopamine receptors. However, few presently available drugs have been proved conclusively to be more effective, overall, than chlorpromazine, and therapeutic advantages have been minimal. With a good battery of predictive animal tests for typical antipsychotics, it has been possible to discover many chemicals with similar properties, but few really new drugs. The release of clozapine will mark the first new antipsychotic drug to be introduced to the United States market in more than a dozen years.

# SCHIZOPHRENIA

## Nature of the Disorder

Despite a great amount of research done by highly competent persons from many disciplines, schizophrenia remains as much a scientific mystery and a personal disaster as ever. One must still call it a disorder, rather than a disease, because its etiology is so uncertain. Indeed, whether schizophrenia represents a single disorder or a syndrome whose clinical manifestations represent multiple disorders of differing pathogenesis remains uncertain.

Descriptive subclassifications of schizophrenia abound. One that has stood the test of time rather well differentiates patients into those with *true schizophrenia* (also known as *process* or *poor prognosis* schizophrenia) and those with *schizophreniform psychosis* (also known as *"reactive"* or *good prognosis* schizophrenia). The latter condition is characterized by an acute psychosis, often related to some life stress. It generally follows a good premorbid adjustment and often remits completely for long periods (Kolakowska et al., 1985).

A more recent attempt at classification divides schizophrenia into two types: an *organic type* manifested by brain atrophy evidenced by ventricular enlargement on computerized tomographic scans and a *functional* type characterized by a disturbance in dopaminergic neurotransmission. Presumably, the former, organic type is unresponsive to drugs and has a preponderance of "negative" symptoms (affective flattening and poverty of speech), whereas the functional type responds to drugs and has a preponderance of "positive" symptoms (delusions, hallucinations, and positive thought disorder). The idea of progressive atrophy of schizophrenic brains surfaces repeatedly but is not yet borne out by any neuropathologic studies (Stevens, 1988).

Various sets of *research diagnostic criteria* have been proposed to make the clinical diagnosis more accurate. When several such sets of criteria are applied to the same patient, they often disagree considerably in defining the clinical diagnosis of schizophrenia. Although one can agree that any step toward making clinical diagnosis more precise is welcome, one must have reservations about the present state of the art (Overall and Hollister, 1979).

These two difficulties, first in determining whether or not one is dealing with a heterogeneous illness and second in making accurate diagnoses, confound the assessment of the value of antipsychotic drugs. Although few doubt the efficacy of these drugs, at least for some patients, the marked variability in response and the fact that many patients obtain little or no benefit from them raise important issues about their proper use.

## Prevalence

The 6-month prevalence rate for schizophrenia in three urban United States samples ranged from 0.6 to 1.1 percent for schizophrenia and from 0.1 to 0.2 percent for schizophreniform disorders (Myers et al., 1984). Lifetime prevalence rates were 1.0 to 1.9 percent and 0.1 to 0.3 percent, respectively (Robins et al.,

1984). Such estimates are close to those made earlier, which postulated that about 1 to 2 percent of the population was susceptible to developing a schizophrenia-like psychosis at some time in their lives. The comparative rarity of schizophrenia, as well as the fact that most families are disrupted and dispersed, has made it difficult to isolate strongly affected families for genetic studies. Recently, linkage of the syndrome to two restriction fragment length polymorphisms on chromosome 5 has been reported (Sherrington et al., 1988).

The burden of schizophrenia far outweighs its prevalence. The disorder tends to occur early in life and may last an entire lifetime. The cost in economic terms of supporting and treating patients is huge. The cost in personal tragedy, not only for the affected person but also for those close, is incalculable.

## Biochemical/Biologic Pathogenesis

The revolution that followed the introduction of effective drugs for treating schizophrenia changed psychiatric thinking tremendously. Schizophrenia is now viewed by the majority of persons as being biologically determined rather than caused by psychosocial stressors in the environment. A vast number of theories have evolved regarding the etiology and pathogenesis of schizophrenia (Table 5-1). None have been absolutely proven, although some may have been disproven.

The dopaminergic hypothesis, which postulates that for one reason or another dopaminergic activity is increased in the mesolimbic system of the brain, is the bedrock on which drug therapy is founded (McKenna, 1987). Evidence has been circumstantial: Schizophrenia-like disorders have followed use of drugs that work through dopaminergic mechanisms (amphetamine psychosis); all effective antipsychotic drugs seem to act by blocking postsynaptic dopamine receptors; schizophrenia may be aggravated by dopamine precursors, such as levodopa, by dopamine releasers, such as amphetamines, and by dopamine receptor agonists, such as apomorphine. Direct links to a dopaminergic abnormality have been more difficult to establish (Kovelman and Scheibel, 1986). A search still continues for other possible mechanisms of drug action that may elucidate the problem of the biochemical pathogenesis of schizophrenia.

## CHEMICAL TYPES OF ANTIPSYCHOTICS

Many chemical compounds have the pharmacologic properties associated with antipsychotic drugs and have been given generic names, with the hope of eventually being marketed. The number that get to the marketplace is considerably fewer, as the market will support only so many drugs. Furthermore, some compounds are either less effective overall than others or are simply duplicates of existing drugs.

Phenothiazine derivatives, as exemplified by chlorpromazine, were the first major group of antipsychotics. Although phenothiazines are the most numerous antipsychotic drugs on the market, their popularity has been waning in recent

### Table 5-1. Some Biochemical/Biologic Theories of Schizophrenia

**Dopaminergic Overactivity**
　　Overproduction due to deficiency of dopamine-beta-hydroxylase (or conversely,
　　　　underproduction of norepinephrine)
　　Accumulation of dopamine due to deficiency of monoamine oxidase
　　Overactivity secondary to diminished inhibitory input through GABA
　　Increased sensitivity or numbers of dopamine-2 receptors
　　Dopamine "dysregulation"
　　Dopamine-receptor-stimulating autoantibiodies

**Indolealkylamine Abnormalities**
　　*N*-methylation to *N, N*-diethyltryptamine
　　Condensation to hallucinogenic beta-carbolines (harmaline-like) or tryptolines

**Other Catecholamine Abnormalities**
　　Transmethylation of dopamine to 3,4-dimethoxphenethylamine

**Endorphins**
　　Excessive beta-endorphin due to failure of end-product inhibition of synthesis due
　　　　to defective formation of des-tyrosine gamma endorphin
　　Deficiency of beta-endorphin

**Autoimmune Disorders**
　　Antibodies attacking specialized dopamine receptors
　　Antibodies attacking specialized regions of brain

**Virus or Other Infectious Agent**
　　Viral damage during brain development
　　Virus-like agent active in brain throughout life

**Dietary**
　　Gluten sensitivity analogous to nontropical sprue
　　Vitamin B-12 or folic acid deficiency

**Abnormalities of Neuromuscular System**
　　Elevated serum concentrations of muscle creatine phosphokinase
　　Abnormal histology of skeletal muscle
　　Smooth-pursuit eye tracking abnormalities

**Structural and Metabolic Abnormalities in Brain**
　　Brain atrophy CT and MRI scans—variable
　　Diminished metabolism PET scans—variable

**Genetic Predisposition**
　　Concordance 50% monozygotic twins
　　Concordance 20% in first-degree relatives

**Environmental Factors**
　　Stress and emotional factors
　　Brain plasticity
　　Parental influences

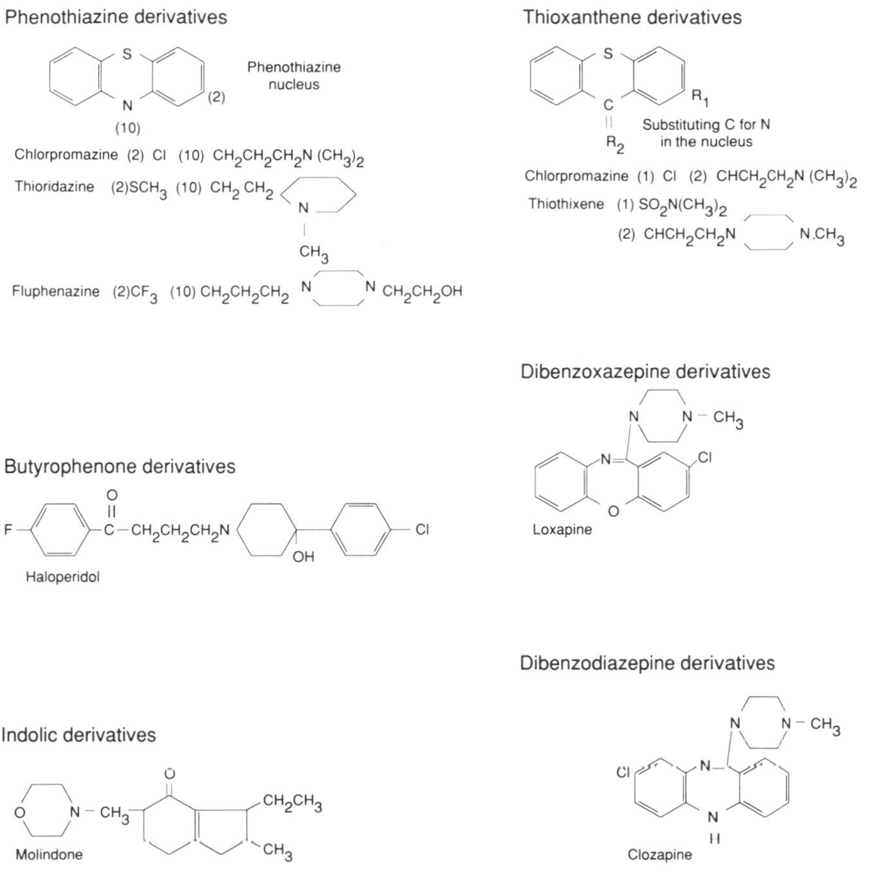

Phenothiazine derivatives

Thioxanthene derivatives

**Fig. 5-1.** Structural formulas for various types of antipsychotic drugs.

years. Three chemical subfamilies can be distinguished based on differences in the side chain (Fig. 5-1). The aliphatic series (exemplified by chlorpromazine) and the piperidine series (exemplified by thioridazine) are generally regarded as low potency compounds, the daily therapeutic doses being measured in hundreds of milligrams. Two variants of the piperazine side chain, along with variations in the ring substituent, create the group of piperazinyl phenothiazines (exemplified by fluphenazine). These compounds are high-potency drugs, the usual daily therapeutic dose being measured in tens of milligrams.

Modification in the ring of the thioxanthenes tends to make for a less potent group of compounds than that of the piperazinyl phenothiazines. The slight loss of potency from the ring structure can be compensated for by the choice of ring substituents and side chains. The dimethylsulfonamide ring substituent and piperazine side chain of thiothixene make it a fairly potent drug.

A number of butyrophenones and the closely related diphenyl-butylpiperidine derivatives have been synthesized and tested for their antipsychotic properties. Haloperidol, now the most often prescribed antipsychotic in the United States, is the only example of these groups that is marketed as an antipsychotic. Others, such as droperidol, are marketed for other indications.

Besides these classes of antipsychotic drugs, three other groups are also represented on the U.S. market: dibenzoxazepines, exemplified by loxitane; indolic derivatives, exemplified by molindone, and dibenzodiazepine derivatives, exemplified by clozapine.

## PHARMACOLOGIC AND BIOCHEMICAL ACTIONS

Several pharmacologic actions in animals are shared by most antipsychotics: (1) inhibition of apomorphine-induced vomiting in dogs; (2) inhibition of apomorphine- or amphetamine-induced stereotyped behaviors in rats; (3) inhibition of conditioned avoidance reactions; (4) production of catalepsy; and (5) inhibition of intracranial self-stimulation. However, the various compounds show enormous differences in potency regarding these tests.

These pharmacologic properties, as well as their biochemical actions, suggest that these drugs are all central dopamine antagonists (Niemegeers and Janssen, 1979). It is believed that postsynaptic receptor blockade in the mesolimbic system of the brain results in the desired therapeutic effect: amelioration of schizophrenic symptoms. Blockade of dopamine receptors in the nigrostriatal dopamine pathway produces an unwanted effect: the extrapyramidal motor reactions.

Recently it has become possible, using PET scanning and suitable radioligands for dopamine-2 receptors, to visualize the binding of ligands to receptors and to estimate the degree of blockade produced by antipsychotics in humans. Clinical doses of all currently used classes of antipsychotics caused a substantial blockade of central dopamine-2 receptors, ranging from 65 to 85 percent occupancy. The degree of blockade persisted for many hours after drugs were stopped and tended to correlate with prevailing plasma concentrations. No such blockade was demonstrated for the tricyclic antidepressant nortriptyline (Farde et al., 1988).

## METABOLISM AND KINETICS

The metabolism and kinetics of chlorpromazine have been most extensively studied, both because it is the prototypic drug and because of the substantial doses used, making measurement in biologic fluids easier. More than 160 metabolites of chlorpromazine are postulated, of which only a minority are identified and still fewer tested for pharmacologic activity. A 7-hydroxy metabolite has activity, but its clinical importance is uncertain. Others may also show minor degrees of activity.

The thiomethyl ring substituent of thioridazine undergoes two sulfoxidations: the sulfoxide (one oxygen) and the sulfone (two oxygen atoms) forms. Both are active metabolites. The sulfoxide and sulfone metabolites are used as separate antipsychotic drugs. Mesoridazine is the sulfoxide, and sulphoridazine is the sulfone. With two active metabolites as well as the parent drug, study of kinetics of this drug, and the relationship of plasma concentrations to clinical efficacy, is difficult.

The metabolism of the piperazinyl phenothiazines is similar to that of chlorpromazine, but to date no active metabolites have been identified. The same is true for thiothixene. The metabolism of haloperidol involves *N*-dealkylation, oxidation, and conjugation. Although an active hydroxy metabolite is formed, its role in the action of the drug is still unsettled.

The kinetics of the various antipsychotics vary, but they share a similar pattern. Most of them are readily but incompletely absorbed, with bioavailability ranging from about 25 to 35 percent for chlorpromazine to about 65 percent for haloperidol (Holley et al., 1983). Protein binding is high, generally in the range of 90 percent. Distribution due to their lipid solubility is great, with all having relatively high apparent volumes of distribution. The elimination half-lives vary in the range of 10 to 24 hours. Very little unchanged drug is excreted; most is nearly totally metabolized.

Now that it is technically possible to measure plasma concentrations of most antipsychotic drugs, a great deal of effort has been expended during the past decade in trying to relate clinical response to antipsychotics with plasma levels of these drugs. What one can say with much assurance is limited, because for virtually every study purporting to show such a relationship, another has failed. Table 5-2 summarizes suggested therapeutic ranges for several commonly used drugs. Haloperidol has been most studied, and there seems to be more general agreement about its therapeutic plasma concentrations than with most others. Still, a range of from 4 to 20 mg/ml is so wide that one wonders how much help measurements of plasma concentrations may be in clinical practice. Thus far, few clinicians feel constrained to obtain such measurements routinely.

**Table 5-2.** Suggested Therapeutic Ranges of Plasma Concentrations of Various Antipsychotics

| Drug | Range (ng/ml) | Reference |
|---|---|---|
| Chlorpromazine | 30–100 | Dahl, 1986 |
| | 50–300 | Rivera-Calimlin, 1976 |
| Perphenazine | 0.8–2.4 | Hanson and Larsen, 1985 |
| Thiothixene | 2–15 | Mavroidis et al., 1984 |
| Fluphenazine | 0.2–2.8 | Baldessarini et al., 1988 |
| Haloperidol | 4.2–11 | Mavroidis et al., 1983 |
| | 8–18 | Magliozzi et al., 1981 |
| | 5–16 | Van Putten et al., 1985 |
| | 10–20 | Zohar et al., 1986 |

# CLINICAL USE OF ANTIPSYCHOTICS
## Indications

### Schizophrenia

The principal indications for use of antipsychotics are summarized in Table 5-3. Although indications are numerous, the treatment of schizophrenia accounts for the vast majority of prescriptions. Schizophrenic patients who do not respond to drug therapy constitute a major problem. One postulate is that they represent "organic" schizophrenia. These patients are often chronically treated and with higher doses of neuroleptics; thus they may be more vulnerable to develop tardive dyskinesia as a long-term complication of drug therapy.

Some types of schizophrenia are self-limited. These "good prognosis" patients may derive some benefit from drug therapy but may do well without it. As it is often difficult to determine whether a patient belongs in this category, most clinicians now believe that a trial without drugs is warranted in all patients who show a good response to drug therapy during their first episode of schizophrenia.

### Schizoaffective Disorders

The "schizo" component of schizoaffective disorders may respond to antipsychotics, but the "affective" component, if it is depression, may require concomitant use of an antidepressant. This disorder is sometimes difficult to distinguish from delusional or psychotic depression, or even schizophrenia with superimposed depression. In any case, the concurrence of both psychosis and

**Table 5-3.** Indications for Antipsychotics

| Firm Indications | |
| --- | --- |
| Schizophrenia | Virtually all types, all stages of the disorder; may be combined with a variety of other psychotherapeutic drugs |
| Schizoaffective disorders | May be combined with antidepressants and/or lithium |
| Mania | Preferred drugs for acute phases; also with lithium |
| Psychosis associated with old age | Symptomatic treatment |
| Tourette syndrome | Most experience with haloperidol |
| Doubtful Indications | |
| Depression | Useful in agitated or psychotic depressions; doubtful utility in pure depression |
| Acute brain syndromes | Generally not drugs of choice for drug withdrawal syndromes; may be needed if psychosis is long-lasting; useful in "recovery room" psychosis |
| Minor emotional disorders | Antianxiety drugs are preferred |

depression is an indication for combined use of an antipsychotic and an antidepressant. Such combinations are best made extemporaneously, using more of one or the other drug depending on the importance of the respective symptoms.

## Catatonia

Although catatonia is most often associated with schizophrenia, it may occur independently. Although far less common than in the era before antipsychotics, it is not rare. Parenteral doses of high potency antipsychotic drugs should probably be the first treatment. In the older literature, barbiturates were thought to be effective. More recently, interest in using benzodiazepines has been stimulated by the availability of effective intramuscular dosage forms of lorazepam and midazolam. ECT is a last-resort treatment, to be used when the patient is unresponsive and deteriorating physically.

## Mania

In many parts of the world, antipsychotics, rather than lithium, are used for managing manic patients, lithium being considered a "mood stabilizer." The relatively slow onset of action of lithium in curbing mania is also a disadvantage in highly agitated manic patients. Nonmanic excited states may also be managed by antipsychotics or by droperidol, a butyrophenone derivative with a much shorter half-life than haloperidol.

## Psychoses of Old Age

Little can be done for patients with Alzheimer's disease, but antipsychotic drugs may curb disturbed behavior, reestablish normal sleep–wake cycles, and possibly enhance self-care. Although relief is purely symptomatic, it may make life more tolerable not only for the patients but also for those who care for them. Thioridazine, because it is less likely than other antipsychotics to evoke extrapyramidal reactions, has been the preferred drug. However, this advantage must be traded off against its potent anticholinergic action, which may lead to increased confusion, as well as a greater alpha-adrenergic blockade, which could lead to orthostatic hypotension.

Other organic psychoses, if they are manifested by severe behavioral symptoms, may require antipsychotics.

## Tourette Syndrome

Tourette syndrome may be less rare than previously believed. Haloperidol is extensively used, but pimozide has been specifically approved for this indication. Recent work suggests that clonidine is also effective. The unpredictable barking tic and outbursts of foul language that these patients suffer are socially disabling and clearly warrant treatment with drugs. Effective doses of antipsychotics may be less than required for treating schizophrenia.

# Doubtful Indications

## Depression

Although some antipsychotic drugs have approved indications for treatment of depression (thioridazine and flupenthixol), the use of these drugs remains controversial. Arguments against their use are: they will probably make truly endogenous depressions worse; they are not necessarily more effective than a placebo, antianxiety drugs, or the sedative tricyclic antidepressants in treating the mixed anxiety and depression so often associated with reactive depressions; and the risk of tardive dyskinesia is too great under these conditions. Some patients undoubtedly are helped more by these drugs than by any others, but antipsychotic drugs are not a preferred treatment.

## Acute Brain Syndromes

Acute brain syndromes due to withdrawal from alcohol or other drugs are best treated by replacing the abused drug with one that is pharmacologically equivalent. Such is clearly not the case with antipsychotic drugs, which are contraindicated. Acute disorders associated with hallucinogenic drugs are usually self-limiting and respond better to antianxiety drugs or conventional sedatives. Antipsychotic drugs may produce effects in these otherwise normal persons that are more disabling than the disorder being treated. When a schizophrenic-like psychosis is precipitated by hallucinogenic drugs, antipsychotic drugs may be indicated, but this situation is usually not evident for several days. Toxicity from amphetamines may be treated with haloperidol, but one must be certain of the identity of the drug overdose. Acute brain syndromes associated with being placed in recovery rooms, coronary care units, or other strange medical surroundings seem to respond better to potent antipsychotics, such as haloperidol, than to conventional sedatives, which often aggravate the delirium.

## Minor Emotional Disorders

Disorders associated with anxiety respond preferentially to antianxiety drugs, which are considerably safer than antipsychotics. Instances of tardive dyskinesia have occurred when even small doses of antipsychotic drugs have been used for such disorders.

Patients with anxiety disorders and a history of drug abuse would now be preferentially treated with buspirone rather than any of the sedative-autonomic group of drugs, including antipsychotics.

# Choice of Drug

Although it has been apparent that some patients respond to one drug but not to another, extensive studies aimed at determining the characteristics of patients who might respond selectively to specific drugs have been generally unrewarding. Differences in response may be mediated more by individual differences among patients than by differences among the drugs.

To choose one drug from a bewildering array of available antipsychotics for initial use in a given patient, learn to use a few drugs well rather than all poorly. A rational way to narrow the choice is to master one of each of the three types of phenothiazines and one of each of the remaining chemical classes of drugs. A possible selection, based on drugs currently available in the United States, is shown in Table 5-4. A basic assumption in making these choices is that differences within a chemical class are less than differences among classes; this suggests the choice of only a single drug in each class.

The best guide to selecting the right drug for individual patients is their past response to a drug. Tolerance for the side effects of various drugs may vary considerably. Some patients are considerably distressed by disturbances of sexual function associated with thioridazine. Others prefer that drug, with its paucity of extrapyramidal reactions, to haloperidol, which is likely to produce many more extrapyramidal reactions.

## Doses

Therapeutic margins for antipsychotic drugs are so wide that a remarkable range of doses have been used (Table 5-5). During the past several years, largely based on a desire to reduce the total exposure to these drugs and avoid tardive dyskinesia, doses have become more conservative, both for initial treatment as

**Table 5-4.** Bases of Choice Among a Limited Number of Antipsychotics

| Drug Type | Drug | Advantages | Disadvantages |
|---|---|---|---|
| Phenothiazines | | | |
| Aliphatic | Chlorpromazine | Inexpensive, fewer movement disorders (Parkinson syndrome, dystonia) | Many side effects virtually unique to it; obsolete; parenteral form irritating |
| Piperidine | Thioridazine | Fewer movement disorders | No parenteral form; 800 mg/day maximal limit; retrograde ejaculation |
| Piperazine | Fluphenazine | Depot and parenteral form | ? increased tardive dyskinesia and acute movement disorders |
| Thioxanthenes | Thiothixene | Parenteral form | |
| Butyrophenone | Haloperidol | Parenteral form | More movement disorders |
| Dibenzoxazepine | Loxapine | Uncertain | |
| Dihydroindolone | Molindone | Less weight gain | |

From Hollister LE (1970), with permission.

**Table 5-5.** Dose Equivalents and Ranges for Various Antipsychotics

| Generic/Trade Names | Relative Potency | Dose Ranges/Day (mg) |
|---|---|---|
| Phenothiazines | | |
| Aliphatic | | |
| Chlorpromazine (Thorazine) | 100 | 50–2000 |
| Piperidine | | |
| Thioridazine (Mellaril) | 100 | 50–800 |
| Mesoridazine (Serentil) | 50 | 25–400 |
| Piperacetazine (Quide) | 10 | 10–160 |
| Piperazine | | |
| Perphenazine (Trilafon) | 10 | 8–64 |
| Trifluoperazine (Stelazine) | 5 | 4–60 |
| Fluphenazine (Prolixin) | 2–3 | 2–60 |
| Thioxanthene | | |
| Thiothixene (Navane) | 2–4 | 6–120 |
| Butyrophenone | | |
| Haloperidol (Haldol) | 2 | 2–100 |
| Dibenzoxazepine | | |
| Loxapine (Loxitane) | 10 | 15–160 |
| Dihydroindolone | | |
| Molindone (Moban) | 10 | 15–225 |
| Dibenzodiazepine | | |
| Clozapine (Clozaril) | 50 | 25–400 |

Modified from Hollister LE (1973), with permission.

well as for maintenance (Baldessarini et al., 1988). Previous attempts to hasten the response of patients by large initial doses ("rapid neuroleptidization") were largely fruitless; this practice has been abandoned.

Acute psychotic patients may require initial doses of 10–20 mg/day of haloperidol or equivalent doses of other drugs. The doses may be augmented if behavioral control is not attained or may be lowered as soon as it is. After stabilization at some optimal dose, attempts should be made to gradually reduce the dose to maintenance levels. How vigorously to treat patients will depend on many factors, the most important being the dose previously required to treat the patient optimally.

A few studies indicate that some treatment-resistant patients may respond to higher than usual doses of antipsychotics. Doses of thiothixene of 120 to 400 mg/day have been used with some success in such patients (Kim and Hollister, 1984). Such treatment should obviously be done with care and be brief. Selection of patients is most important, as routine use of high doses will certainly overtreat many patients.

Another potentially useful approach to treatment-resistant patients has been the use of clozapine. More than 300 schizophrenic patients who had failed to respond to at least three different antipsychotics, including a 6-week course of haloperidol 60 mg/day with benztropine mesylate, were randomly assigned to treatment with clozapine (up to 900 mg/day) or chlorpromazine (up to 1800 mg/day) with benztropine mesylate. Only 3 percent improved with haloperidol, and 5 percent with chlorpromazine, but 34 percent of these refractory patients improved with clozapine (Kane et al., 1988). In another study of 34 patients with either treatment resistance or neurologic side effects, clozapine was effective. Thirteen were improved with subsidence of the previous neurologic complications. Effective doses ranged between 270 and 325 mg/day (Small et al., 1987).

Giving initial doses of drugs intramuscularly is a practice recently revived; it was the standard way of initiating treatment when chlorpromazine and reserpine were first introduced. Advantages are that one is absolutely certain of getting the drug into the body and the feedback of clinical effects is prompt. After a few doses given in this fashion, the usual practice is to switch to oral medication, which suffices for most patients. Doses of oral drug may have to be greater than the intramuscular doses by a factor of two or more to be equivalent.

## Dosage Schedules

Divided doses of drug are desirable for rapid titration of dose and assessment of potential side effects. An initial dose of drug may be small, to test the patient's response to it. One or two hours following an intramuscular test dose or 2 to 3 hours following an oral test dose, the degree of sedation and other side effects can be assessed. If the first dose was well-tolerated, doses of this size are then given twice or three times a day to achieve the chosen daily dose. A gradual response of the patient over several days should be expected. Occasional extra doses of neuroleptic or an alternative sedative (e.g., benzodiazepine) may be used for control of behavioral agitation. Frequency of dose should be reduced once it is clear the patient tolerates the drug and the clinical response is apparent. The goal is a single daily dose to be given in the evening; this practice assists sleep while avoiding excessive daytime sedation. Also, patients are less likely to suffer disabling extrapyramidal symptoms if the major impact of the drug occurs while they are sleeping. Manifestations of Parkinson's disease are ameliorated by sleep, for reasons still not clear. Usually a single evening dose is feasible. Many drugs are now available in larger single-dose units to meet the growing acceptance of the single daily dose.

## Maintenance Treatment

Except for those patients who fall into the good prognosis category, the majority of schizophrenics will require some kind of management for an entire lifetime. It is a reasonable custom to gradually withdraw all drugs in patients after their first episode of schizophrenia so as to determine, by the rate and severity of relapse, which patients may require continuing treatment.

Even when it is determined that patients require continued drug treatment, the goal should be to use as little drug as necessary to maintain remission.

Clearly efforts to reduce total exposure to drug therapy are best made during the prolonged maintenance phase rather than during the relatively brief acute treatment phase.

Two somewhat different approaches to reducing exposure to drugs during maintenance treatment have been taken. The first is simply to use the smallest possible dose, but keep the patient constantly under treatment. The second is to use drug therapy on an "as needed" basis, using the early signs of relapse to determine when treatment should be resumed.

The use of low maintenance doses on a continual basis has been explored in several studies. In one study, 94 chronic schizophrenics were divided into a group that continued to receive their usual maintenance dose, a group that had the dose reduced equivalent to 100 mg/day of chlorpromazine, and a third group in whom the dose was further reduced to the equivalent of 50 mg/day of chlorpromazine. The three groups had nonsignificant differences in relapse rates over the following year. Thus, it appeared that even very low oral maintenance dose schedules were effective in preventing relapse (Lehmann et al., 1983). In another study, patients who were already being maintained on a dose of fluphenazine decanoate of 25 mg every 2 weeks were switched in a blind fashion to continuing that dose or having it reduced to 5 mg. After 1 year, relapse rates were the same in both groups (Marder et al., 1984). Other studies have confirmed these observations.

The "as needed" treatment approach has a similar objective but uses a different technique. It requires that patients be under the observation of persons able to spot the earliest symptoms of relapse. After initial treatment with drugs they may be stopped when the patient has reached remission. They may be restarted only when patients show the initial symptoms of relapse (insomnia, irritability, loose thinking). When patients managed in this fashion were compared with those continued on their usual maintenance dose of drugs, they spent only slightly more time in hospital, used considerably fewer drugs, were brighter, and had fewer side effects (Herz, 1985). These studies are continuing.

It would appear to be a matter of choice between the two maintenance programs. Continual treatment with low doses would be the most feasible management of patients with a high rate of previous relapses. In such instances, depot preparations might be preferred to oral dose forms. "As needed" drug therapy might be suitable for patients in aftercare that provides for close and skilled observation by conscientious caretakers and ready access to medical facilities. Thus, the choice of maintenance plans must be made individually for each patient.

## Pharmaceutical Preparations

All antipsychotics are available for oral administration. Many are available as liquid concentrates, which are easier to administer to patients who resist medication. This dosage form is usually more expensive than other oral forms.

The availability of parenteral forms of high potency neuroleptics, such as haloperidol, thiothixene, and fluphenazine, has revived the custom of giving initial doses of these drugs intramuscularly to patients in whom there may be doubt about their willingness to take oral medication. Such routes need only be used briefly, as patients rapidly become more tractable.

Depot preparations of various drugs or hormones for intramuscular administration have long been available. Many of these are fatty acid esters of drugs or hormones that contain an alcohol moiety, $CH_2OH$, so that drug$-CH_2O-$fatty acid becomes the new molecule. This new molecule is attacked by esterases ubiquitous in tissues so that the parent compound is regenerated at a slow rate. Placing the fatty acid esters in a lipid vehicle further slows the release of drug.

A number of such depot preparations of antipsychotic drugs have been used in clinical practice. In the United States, fluphenazine, either as the enanthate or decanoate ester, has been on the market for many years and has enjoyed extensive use. More recently a decanoate ester of haloperidol has been marketed. Studies done before its introduction indicate that patients previously treated with oral antipsychotics can be effectively maintained on the depot preparation and that plasma levels of the drug are comparable to those attained from an equivalent oral dose administered daily (Beresford and Ward, 1987).

The exact place of such depot preparations in treatment is still controversial. No one would argue that they are not useful in treating patients whose dependability for taking oral medication is questionable. As many patients seem to relapse and return to mental hospitals owing to some breach in maintenance drug treatment, such patients are most suitable for depot preparations, which generally need to be given at intervals of 2 to 4 weeks and which can be given at home by visiting nurses. However, they need not be used in the majority of patients. One study, which compared maintenance doses of fluphenazine hydrochloride given orally with fluphenazine decanoate in 290 newly admitted schizophrenics, revealed no difference in the relapse rates during a follow-up period of up to 1 year (Schooler et al., 1980).

## Combinations of Drugs

The most frequently prescribed class of drugs combined with antipsychotics are antiparkinson drugs. Their routine use in all patients for whom antipsychotics are prescribed is unnecessary, as not all patients will develop one of the early extrapyramidal manifestations: Parkinson syndrome, akathisia, or acute dystonia. However, when treating young persons, especially men, who are most prone to developing acute dystonic reactions, one is justified in using antiparkinson drugs prophylactically. This long-standing custom was recently confirmed by a review of the extensive literature (Arana et al., 1988). For other patients, however, it is more appropriate to wait until manifestations of extrapyramidal effects appear. Traditional anticholinergic antiparkinson drugs, such as benztropine and trihexiphenidyl, are used most often. Amantadine may not cause as much cognitive impairment as do anticholinergics, but its cost is somewhat greater and it can occasionally exacerbate psychosis.

No rationale exists for combining two antipsychotic drugs. However, tricyclic antidepressants are often combined with antipsychotics. If the attempt is to allay the social withdrawal and blunted affect of schizophrenic patients, such combinations are not likely to be successful. On the other hand, depressed schizophrenics, or those with schizoaffective disorder with depression, may benefit from such a combination. So might many agitated or psychotically depressed patients, for whom the antipsychotic is added to treatment with the antidepressant.

Lithium or carbamazepine is often added when patients do not respond adequately to antipsychotics. Although largely based on empiric observations, the effects are often appreciable. Whether such patients represent instances of mania misdiagnosed as schizophrenia or whether lithium and carbamazepine may have some direct, though weaker, antipsychotic action is still uncertain. One should be aware that lithium tends to exacerbate the extrapyramidal motor reactions produced by antipsychotics.

Before the advent of antipsychotic drugs, treatment of agitated or assaultive behavior relied exclusively on barbiturates, usually amobarbital sodium given intramuscularly or intravenously. Following the introduction of chlorpromazine, its use intramuscularly was effective, but pain at the site of intramuscular injection and hypotension were limiting factors in its use. A combination of 100 mg chlorpromazine and 130 mg phenobarbital sodium often avoided the need for repeated doses, establishing the principle of combining an antipsychotic and a sedative–hypnotic (Hollister, 1973). Haloperidol and other high-potency neuroleptics that were well tolerated after intramuscular injection replaced chlorpromazine. However, not until the advent of a reliably absorbed intramuscular form of lorazepam was it possible to replace the barbiturate with a benzodiazepine in such combinations.

The combination most preferred is haloperidol and lorazepam intramuscularly. When this combination was compared with haloperidol alone for treating agitated patients, 50 percent less dosage of the antipsychotic was required (Salzman et al., 1986). Tremendously high doses of the combination (100–480 mg of haloperidol and 36–480 mg of lorazepam) have been used for treating organic delirium in critically ill cancer patients (Adams et al., 1986). If nothing else, this study testifies to the safety of the two drugs. One must assume that sedative–hypnotics are used in this situation simply for that effect and not for any specific antipsychotic action.

Anxiety or insomnia unrelieved by antipsychotic drugs, or even possibly aggravated by them, might require the addition of a benzodiazepine. The same basic principle applies to this use of benzodiazepines as applies to their use in nonpsychotic patients: One wishes to limit the time and amount of drug to the greatest extent possible.

# NEW DEVELOPMENTS IN ANTIPSYCHOTICS
## Atypical Antipsychotics

Clozapine, an atypical neuroleptic, may not produce tardive dyskinesia. Unfortunately, it has several disadvantages, not the least of which was the production of the greatest epidemic of drug-induced agranulocytosis in medical history. Despite that drawback, which may have represented an unusual situation, the drug can be used under very close control in otherwise refractory patients or in those who may be disabled by tardive dyskinesia. The potential advantage of having a drug that does not evoke extrapyramidal syndromes, perhaps by favoring the mesolimbic dopamine system as the site of action, has impelled much research toward discovering such new agents. Some have attributed the atypical properties of clozapine to its antagonist action at serotonin-5HT-2 or dopamine-D-1 receptors.

## New Butyrophenones and Diphenylbutylpiperdines

Bromperidol, which is chemically similar to haloperidol, has been extensively studied (Benfield et al., 1988). Although there is no reason to believe that this drug is not as active as haloperidol, whether it has any advantage over the latter drug is questionable. This drug will probably not be introduced in the United States. Tiaspirone, an analog of buspirone, has shown some efficacy in schizophrenics and produced no extrapyramidal syndromes. Abnormal hepatic tests could be a major problem with this drug (Moore et al., 1987).

## Benzamides

This class of drugs has some members with antipsychotic actions. Presumably they have fewer extrapyramidal side effects than older antipsychotics. Sulpiride has been the most studied. Although it has been thought to be as effective as other antipsychotics, its promise of few extrapyramidal actions may be illusory. Remoxipride and raclopride have just begun to be studied in schizophrenic patients; early studies suggest some degree of efficacy with relatively few side effects (Laursen and Gerlach, 1986). The benzamides have been somewhat controversial, because of antipsychotic actions that are less than desirable or extrapyramidal side effects that are more than anticipated.

## New Uses for Other Types of Drug

Almost 20 years after the first use of propranolol in schizophrenics, it is difficult to say just how effective the drug is. A placebo-controlled trial of propranolol in 36 acute schizophrenics showed a barely detectable clinical effect (Mandhanda and Hirsch, 1986). A trial of propranolol as an adjunct for treatment-resistant patients indicated more improvement than from addition of placebo, but it was less dramatic than earlier reports. The authors called attention to the possibility of a pharmacokinetic interaction, in which propranolol might augment plasma concentrations of concurrently used neuroleptics (Pugh et al., 1983). Propranolol has also gained a reputation as being an effective adjunct for aggressive patients. Despite the high doses used, the drug appears to be safe. Whether the mechanism of improvement is due to beta-receptor blockade, a membrane-stabilizing action, or simply additional sedation is not clear.

Although benzodiazepines have never been considered as potential antipsychotic drugs, the notion that they may diminish dopaminergic activity when given in high doses has stimulated some new interest in using them for treating schizophrenia. Although little reason has been adduced to use these drugs as antipsychotics, benzodiazepines may "spare" antipsychotics so that less of the latter drugs can be used. Clonazepam was added to existing antipsychotic drugs in doses of 3 to 4 mg/day in 13 schizophrenics. Aggressive behavior was diminished in four patients, consistent with the sedative actions of the drug, but no specific antipsychotic effects were observed (Karson et al., 1982).

Clonidine was first tried for treating schizophrenics in the mid-1960s and was found to be ineffective. No reason exists to change that conclusion despite a recent revival of interest in the drug. Dopamine agonists, such as apomorphine and bromocriptine, may act at dopamine autoreceptors to inhibit release and have been alleged to be effective. Such reports have been difficult to confirm. Several partial dopamine agonists have now been developed; no doubt they will be assessed for antipsychotic action as well. Naloxone and opioid peptides as treatments for schizophrenia engendered a burgeoning literature that is best forgotten. The same is true for other neuropeptides, such as the cholecystokinin homolog, ceruletide.

## SIDE EFFECTS AND COMPLICATIONS

Adverse reactions to drugs can generally be placed in three major categories: extensions of known and expected pharmacologic effects of the drug (although sometimes in novel and unexpected ways); allergic or hypersensitivity reactions; and those of known or unknown mechanisms that are peculiar (idiosyncratic) to a patient.

Reactions to psychotherapeutic drugs have been of great interest because some have provided remarkably good models for naturally occurring illnesses. The amine hypothesis for endogenous depressions emanated from the observation that reserpine made patients depressed. The use of levodopa as a treatment for Parkinson's disease evolved after the model of this illness produced by antipsychotic drugs was fully investigated. Tardive dyskinesia bears some resemblance to Huntington's disease. Even our understanding of the disorders we treat, whose cause is generally unknown, has been enhanced by study of both the wanted and unwanted effects of drugs.

Some of the unwanted effects of these drugs that are mediated by their pharmacologic actions are shown in Table 5-6. The majority of side effects of antipsychotic drugs are due to extensions of their known pharmacologic actions.

### Adverse Behavioral Effects

Of greatest concern is the possibility that long-term treatment with antipsychotics may induce supersensitivity of dopamine receptors in the mesolimbic system with the need for increasing doses to maintain the antipsychotic effect. This apparent "tolerance" may be associated with *dependence*, in the sense that on withdrawal of neuroleptics, symptoms may be worse than before treatment.

**Table 5-6.** Unwanted Pharmacologic Effects of Antipsychotic Drugs

| Type | Manifestation | Mechanism |
|---|---|---|
| Adverse behavioral effects | Excitement, akinesia | Dopamine receptor blockade |
| | Supersensitivity psychosis | Denervation supersensitivity from block of dopamine receptors |
| | Toxic-confusional state | Block of muscarinic cholinergic receptors |
| Neurologic | Parkinson syndrome, akathisia, dystonias | Dopamine receptor blockade |
| | Tardive dyskinesia | Supersensitivity of receptors |
| Autonomic nervous system | Blurred vision, dry mouth, urinary hesitancy, constipation | Block of muscarinic cholinergic receptors |
| | Orthostatic hypotension, impotence, failure to ejaculate | Alpha-adrenoreceptor blockade |
| Metabolic-endocrine | Amenorrhea-galactorrhea, infertility, impotence | Dopamine receptor block in tuberoinfundibular tract |
| Others | Heat stroke, neuroleptic malignant syndrome | Loss of central control of body temperature |
| | Cardiac toxicity | Quinidine-like actions on membranes |

This phenomenon is called *neuroleptic-induced supersensitivity psychosis.* Evidence for such a phenomenon is primarily based on an analogy with tardive dyskinesia (dopaminergic supersensitivity in the nigrostriatal pathway as opposed to the mesolimbic system) and supported by clinical anecdote. The evidence overall is that some such condition exists, although it seems to be relatively uncommon (Jain et al., 1988). The possible occurrence of supersensitivity psychosis is still another reason for not using more antipsychotic drug than is absolutely needed.

## Adverse Neurologic Effects

The Parkinson syndrome, akathisia, and acute dystonic reactions are well-recognized and frequent neurologic consequences of antipsychotic drugs. Seldom do they necessitate abandonment of treatment, as they are generally easily managed. Traditional anticholinergic antiparkinson drugs have been most widely used for treatment, but amantadine has also been used with probably less cognitive impairment. Akathisia has been managed effectively with a drug such as diphenhydramine, which has both anticholinergic and sedative properties. Recently, propranolol and other beta-adrenoreceptor blocking drugs have also been used with benefit (Dupuis et al., 1987). Clonidine has also been said to be effective, possibly by nonspecific sedative effects. Acute dystonia occurs mainly in men (about two-thirds of cases) and is rare in patients over 40 years of age (Keepers and Casey, 1987).

The concept of tardive dyskinesia has been broadened, but the most frequent manifestation is repetitive involuntary movements of a choreoathetoid type involving the mouth, tongue, neck, trunk, and extremities. Although spontaneous orofacial dyskinesias may occur in elderly patients who have never received antipsychotics, little doubt exists that tardive dyskinesia of the classic type is a consequence of drug therapy. In addition to this most prevalent type, five other variants have been described: tardive limb dyskinesia, tardive dystonia, tardive Tourette syndrome, tardive dysmentia, and tardive akathisia (Stahl, 1986). Tardive dystonia may resemble spastic torticollis or be manifested primarily by blepharospasm. Unlike classic tardive dyskinesia, it is rarely reversible.

Prevalence rates vary widely, depending on the population studied. Current estimates are that 20 to 40 percent of chronically hospitalized schizophrenics develop tardive dyskinesia, but the rate is less when all patients exposed to antipsychotics are considered. Predisposing factors have varied; increasing age has been found to be a predisposing factor in virtually every study. Women have been found to be more often affected than men, although the reverse situation has been described (Morgenstern et al., 1987). Duration of exposure to drugs, exposure to depot preparations, and frequency of drug-free periods have also been considered as predisposing (Branchey and Branchey, 1984). Thus, efforts to forestall the development of tardive dyskinesia by interruptions in treatment may be misdirected.

Although the dopamine receptor supersensitivity hypothesis of the pathogenesis of this disorder has been challenged, it still makes considerable sense and explains a number of clinical phenomena: aggravation of the syndrome when antipsychotics are abruptly discontinued; relief of symptoms by increased doses of antipsychotics; worsening when anticholinergic antiparkinson drugs are used for treatment. Denervation supersensitivity of receptors via drug blockade seems to have emerged as a general rule in a variety of neurotransmitter systems. If this homeostatic mechanism overshoots the mark so that too little dopamine receptor activity initially is converted to too much, tardive dyskinesia might result.

A simplified view of connections between the substantia nigra and the caudate-putamen is shown in Figure 5-2. An inhibitory dopamine neuron in the substantia nigra projects to a short stimulatory cholinergic neuron in the caudate-putamen that in turn synapses with an inhibitory gamma-aminobutyric acid (GABA) neuron that controls the amount of movement. Thus, the relative amount of dopaminergic and cholinergic activity regulates the amount of inhibition of movement exerted by the GABA neuron that projects to the thalamus and pyramidal system. If dopaminergic activity is decreased, as by death of neurons in the substantia nigra in Parkinson's disease, or by postsynaptic block of dopamine receptors, as occurs in the drug-induced Parkinson syndrome, increased GABA inhibition produces decreased total motor movement. Conversely, increased dopaminergic activity, as occurs in tardive dys-

DOPAMINERGIC-CHOLINERGIC
BALANCE IN STRIATUM

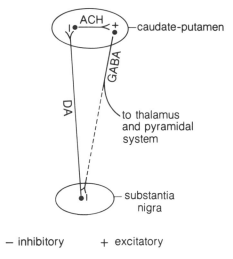

− inhibitory     + excitatory

DA-dopamine; ACH-acetylcholine;

GABA-gamma-aminobutyric acid

**Fig. 5-2.** Schema of control of efferent GABA pathway controlling motor movement. The interplay between the inhibitory actions of dopamine and the excitatory actions of acetylcholine determines the amount of inhibitory GABA output.

kinesia and in levodopa-induced dyskinesia, produces the opposite end result, an increase in motor activity.

Such a scheme suggests three points of pharmacologic attack. Reducing dopaminergic activity would be desirable. The most expeditious way to do this would be to stop antipsychotic drugs and permit supersensitive receptors to become desensitized. Often this approach is not clinically feasible. Reserpine, which depletes stores of neurotransmitters at synapses has been tried, but it has the theoretic disadvantage of possibly aggravating the situation over the long run. Clozapine, a site-selective antipsychotic, may turn out to be the most acceptable method, as treatment with an antipsychotic drug can be continued without worsening of the dyskinesia (Simpson et al., 1986). Another point of attack would be to increase cholinergic activity. Physostigmine is helpful but not easily applied clinically. Attempts to use cholinergic precursors, such as choline and lecithin, have been fruitless. Whether tetrahydroaminacrine, which can be given orally, will be useful remains to be seen. Most important is stopping anticholinergic drugs, most commonly antiparkinson drugs and tricyclic antidepressants. Last, increasing activity of GABA systems is best done with benzodiazepines. Diazepam, clonazepam, and others have been used with some success. High doses may be required, which somewhat limits the acceptability. Diltiazem, as well as verapamil, has been reported to alleviate tardive dyskinesia. Just how calcium channel blockers do this is not certain (Ross et al., 1987).

The key to managing tardive dyskinesia is to prevent it. Conservative use of neuroleptics, close monitoring of patients, and early recognition of the syndrome are important. Early cases are reversible but well-established "grotesques" may not be.

Movement disorders are said to be underdiagnosed. Dyskinesias of the extremities may be masked or considered to be tremors. Severe akinesia may be misdiagnosed as depression and akathisia as psychotic restlessness. New muscle spasms or posturing early during treatment may represent dystonic reactions (Weiden et al., 1987).

## Neuroleptic Malignant Syndrome

This syndrome may best be thought of as a neurologic complication, due to either an acute decrease in dopaminergic activity or an abrupt increase in cholinergic activity with severe extrapyramidal symptoms. The following manifestations are characteristic: (1) changes in consciousness ranging from lethargy and confusion to stupor or coma; (2) extrapyramidal symptoms manifested by increased muscle tone, rigidity, tremor, akinesia, dysarthria, and dysphagia; (3) fever, which may not be present if sweating is preserved; if sweating stops hyperthermia may develop; (4) autonomic instability, manifested by blood pressure changes, tachycardia, and tachypnea; (5) laboratory abnormalities with (a) increased serum creatine phosphokinase and possibly other enzymes, (b) increased serum potassium, associated with muscle damage, (c) leukocytosis associated with dehydration and stress. Incomplete forms of neuroleptic malignant syndrome are being increasingly recognized (Guze and Baxter, 1985).

Current estimates of prevalence are about 1 percent in hospitalized patients (Keck et al., 1987). The clinical course may last a few days, subsiding after withdrawal from antipsychotics and with supportive treatment. Deaths are less frequent now than in the past, but the mortality rate was 11 percent in a recently reported review of 115 case reports (Addonizio et al., 1987). Deaths are usually associated with some complication, such as rhabdomyolysis, disseminated intravascular coagulation, aspiration pneumonia, or cardiopulmonary arrest. Virtually all antipsychotics have been involved, but high potency drugs given parenterally are most commonly associated. Even dopamine receptor blocking drugs not used or thought of as antipsychotics, such as metoclopramide, have been associated with the syndrome (Friedman et al., 1987). Rare reports have implicated lithium or tricyclics. Sudden withdrawal from antiparkinson drugs, such as anticholinergics or levodopa, may also precipitate the syndrome, giving credence to the belief that both sudden dopaminergic and cholinergic changes may cause it.

The presence of high fever and leukocytosis may result in some patients being mistakenly treated for infectious disease with antibiotics. History of use of antipsychotics and the presence of extrapyramidal syndromes should point to the correct diagnosis. Other causes of fever associated with antipsychotics, such as the heat-stroke syndrome (only when ambient temperatures are high) and chlorpromazine jaundice or other allergies, lack the characteristic extrapyramidal syndrome.

Treatment may be directed at peripheral or central mechanisms. Peripheral treatment includes mechanical cooling and the use of skeletal muscle relaxants, such as dantrolene sodium (which may be given IV), baclofen, or diazepam. Central approaches attempt to restore an adequate amount of dopaminergic activity by use of direct agonists, such as bromocriptine, uptake inhibitors, such as amantadine, or precursors, such as levodopa. Electroconvulsive therapy has been effective, for reasons that are unclear.

A state with features of both catatonia and the Parkinson syndrome was reported following neuroleptic treatment in four patients. Two of these patients were probably early in the development of neuroleptic malignant syndrome. Rapid treatment with intravenous doses of lorazepam reversed the situation in all four patients (Frichhione et al., 1983). This experience raises the question of whether early recognition of the syndrome and treatment with intravenous sedatives might forestall full-blown development of neuroleptic malignant syndrome.

## Toxic and Allergic Reactions

Agranulocytosis, a direct toxic action of chlorpromazine on the bone marrow, is extremely rare with the more potent antipsychotics. Although clozapine produced the greatest epidemic of drug-induced agranulocytosis in history, special circumstances, such as concurrent use of dipyrone, a known toxic drug, make this episode atypical. Current prevalence of agranulocytosis with clozapine is estimated to be 3 percent, which means that the drug will have to be used with close clinical and laboratory monitoring. Cholestatic jaundice is now rare because chlorpromazine is seldom used. Rashes are seldom major problems with any antipsychotic.

## Autonomic Nervous System Effects

Blurred vision, dry mouth, difficulty in urinating, and constipation are the most frequent anticholinergic effects. These symptoms are usually simply bothersome. The sympatholytic actions of these drugs may produce orthostatic hypotension or acute hypotensive crises, especially in old or debilitated patients. Chlorpromazine and thioridazine are the worst offenders. The latter drug has such strong alpha-adrenergic receptor blocking actions that ejaculation may be inhibited.

## Metabolic and Endocrine Effects

Weight gain, due to both increased appetite and decreased activity, may be substantial and troublesome. Not all neuroleptics cause increased weight; both molindone and loxapine may cause weight loss. Whether such loss is due to a direct anorexigenic effect, an increase in nausea, or to increased activity is still uncertain (Gardos and Cole, 1977).

Galactorrhea, accompanied by amenorrhea, is observed commonly in women treated chronically with antipsychotics and is due to increased circulating levels of prolactin, secondary to suppression of release of dopamine blockade, the prolactin-inhibiting factor in the pituitary. Patients with amenorrhea tend to show variable concentrations of luteinizing hormone (LH) with absent midcycle peaks. Thus, failure to menstruate may be attributable to a loss of the cyclic tide of LH, estradiol, and progesterone.

Hyperprolactinemia in men is associated with decreased libido, impotence, and sterility. It is not surprising that drugs that increase levels of prolactin, such as most antipsychotics, also impair male sexual function. In addition, drugs with strong anticholinergic effects can interfere with erection. Naturally, such problems are more frequent with drugs that have strong anticholinergic actions such as thioridazine. It is very likely schizophrenic patients have a less than normally active sexual life and the drugs used in their treatment make it worse. Although there has been some concern about development of breast cancers from long-standing hyperprolactinemia, retrospective studies indicate no such increase among patients treated with antipsychotics.

The syndrome of inappropriate secretion of antidiuretic hormone can be induced by a number of antipsychotic drugs, including thioridazine, haloperidol, thiothixene, and fluphenazine. However, this syndrome as well as psychogenic polydipsia can also be found in psychiatric patients who are taking no drugs (Smith and Clark, 1980). Accordingly, it is difficult to determine the exact role of drugs in this syndrome.

## Ocular Complications

Granular deposits in the cornea and lens occur in about 20 to 30 percent of patients treated with long-term chloropromazine; this complication is somewhat dose-related. Such changes seldom lead to loss of visual acuity. More serious is the pigmentary retinopathy associated with thioridazine. The clinical picture begins with deposits of dark pigment surrounding the macula, the "bull's-eye" lesion, that eventually may extend throughout the entire retina and resemble retinitis pigmentosa (Meredith et al., 1978).

## Cardiac Toxicity and Sudden Death

Abnormal T-waves, sometimes with prolonged ventricular repolarization, can be observed almost routinely in electrocardiograms (ECGs) of patients on substantial doses of thioridazine, mesoridazine, and, to a lesser extent, those on other antipsychotic drugs. It is reversible, and the significance of this "disorder" remains controversial. Regardless of its cause, any increase in ventricular repolarization enhances the likelihood of re-entry rhythms. Ventricular tachycardia has been well documented as one of the potentially life-threatening arrhythmias that may be induced by phenothiazines, especially thioridazine, and tricyclics, especially amitriptyline. Such life-threatening arrhythmias may occur on therapeutic as well as suicidal doses of these drugs (Fowler et al., 1976). Although the cardiac toxicity of thioridazine in therapeutic doses has been debatable, there is now little doubt about its severe cardiac effects when taken in overdose. Six cases, five of which were fatal, were tracked down in a relatively small community over a relatively short time period. Four patients did not reach the hospital alive, as their deaths occurred too quickly for medical intervention (Donlon and Tupin, 1977). Formerly, it was generally believed that overdoses of phenothiazines were rarely fatal. Increased QT intervals are also seen with pimozide, a neuroleptic most often used in children to treat Tourette syndrome.

A critical issue is whether or not sudden (within seconds or minutes), unexpected (no known antecedents), and unexplained (no plausible postmortem explanation) deaths are associated with antipsychotic drug treatment. This issue was recently reviewed at length without any definite conclusion being drawn (Lathers and Lipka, 1987). The American Psychiatric Association set up a special task force to review the evidence, and they, too, found it difficult to prove or to deny such an association (APA Task Force, 1988). Even if an association were established, it is impossible to predict in advance which patients are at greatest risk or how such fatalities might be prevented. Episodes of unexplained blackouts or faints during treatment should call for monitoring of cardiac rhythm.

## INTERACTIONS

### Pharmacodynamic

The most important pharmacodynamic interaction of neuroleptics is with various other central nervous system depressants in which an additive depressant effect is obtained. Such drugs include conventional sedatives and hypnotics, antihistamines, opiates, and alcohol.

The anticholinergic effects of various neuroleptics vary in intensity, but they are often used with other drugs, such as antiparkinson agents or tricyclic antidepressants, that are strongly anticholinergic. The onset of delirium in the presence of psychosis may be deceiving so that more drug is added. Peripheral anticholinergic effects are more easily recognized.

The alpha-adrenergic receptor blocking actions of some neuroleptics, especially chlorpromazine and thioridazine, are strong and may produce additive orthostatic hypotensive effects when combined with monoamine oxidase inhibitors. The antidepressant trazodone, which has only mild alpha-adrenergic blocking action, also produced hypotension when added to treatment with phenothiazines (Asayesh, 1986).

Thioridazine has quinidine-like effects that are possibly related to its apparent cardiotoxicity. Other drugs with such actions include quinidine and procainamide, tricyclic antidepressants, and hydroxyzine (Hollister, 1975). The use of thioridazine with any of these types of drugs should be avoided as the arrhythmogenic potential of the drug may be increased.

## Pharmacokinetic

Some neuroleptics have been reported to decrease metabolism and increase plasma concentrations of some tricyclics and vice versa. As doses of both drugs are empirically chosen and the range of effective doses and plasma concentrations is wide, this interaction is probably of little clinical significance. A possible interaction between phenothiazines, specifically thioridazine, and phenytoin might be of greater consequence. Inhibition of metabolism of phenytoin, which has a narrow therapeutic range, has led to serious clinical toxicity (Vincent, 1980).

Two patients taking a standard oral dose of thioridazine showed a three- to five-fold increase in plasma concentrations of the drug when propranolol was added. Neither showed any clinical signs of toxicity despite the fact that their thioridazine and mesoridazine levels were in a potentially toxic range (Silver et al., 1986). The addition of carbamazepine to haloperidol (a fairly common clinical practice) resulted in about a 60 percent decrease in plasma levels of haloperidol over a period of 2 to 3 weeks. No adverse effects were noted, but loss of efficacy might be possible (Jann et al., 1985). For the most part, pharmacokinetic interactions have not been a source of serious trouble.

## OVERDOSE

Symptoms from poisonings with various antipsychotics are similar, probably because the various drugs are similar pharmacologically. Poisonings with phenothiazine derivatives are probably common, yet reports in the literature are scarce. Perhaps this rarity of case reports is due to the almost uniformly favorable outcome. Most fatal cases from ingestion of chlorpromazine are in children. Documented cases of overdoses with thioxanthene derivatives, such as chlorprothixene, again indicate no lethal outcomes. Equivalent doses of thiothixene are probably equally safe. Haloperidol is not associated with any deaths following overdoses, and that may prove the case with other butyrophenones. Thioridazine and mesoridazine may be lethal in overdose owing to production of ventricular tachyarrhythmia.

General principles of management of overdoses apply to phenothiazines, but some special problems are of concern. Convulsions are best treated by intravenous injections of diazepam or sodium phenytoin. The possibility of increasing central respiratory depression with further doses of a central depressant drug should be balanced against the anticonvulsant effect, and only minimally effective doses should be used. Acute hypotension not responsive to forced fluids may require the use of a pressor agent. Norepinephrine is the logical drug for treatment, being primarily an alpha-adrenergic receptor stimulant. Warm blankets and heat cradles may reverse the trend toward hypothermia, but if one overshoots, fever will ensue. Do not ascribe fever to some infectious complication in the absence of other evidence.

# REFERENCES

Adams F, Fernandez F, Anderson B (1986) Emergency pharmacotherapy of delirium in the critically ill cancer patients. Psychosomatics 27:33–37

Addonizio G, Susman VL, Roth SD (1987) Neuroleptic malignant syndrome: Review and analysis of 115 cases. Biol Psychiatry 22:1004–1020

APA Task Force Report (1988) Sudden Death in Psychiatric Patients. TF #27. American Psychiatric Press, Washington, DC

Arana GW, Goff DC, Baldessarini RJ, Keepers GA (1988) Efficacy of anticholinergic prophylaxis for neuroleptic-induced dystonia. Am J Psychiatry 145:993–996

Asayesh K (1986) Combination of trazodone and phenothiazines: a possible additive hypotensive effect. Can J Psychiatry 31:857–858

Baldessarini RJ, Cohen BM, Teicher MH (1988) Significance of neuroleptic dose and plasma level in the pharmacological treatment of psychoses. Arch Gen Psychiatry 45:79–91

Benfield P, Ward A, Clark BG, Jue SG (1988) Bromperidol: a preliminary review of its pharmacodynamic and pharmacokinetic properties, and therapeutic efficacy in psychoses. Drugs 35:670–684

Beresford R, Ward A (1987) Haloperidol decanoate. A preliminary review of its pharmacodynamic and pharmacokinetics properties and therapeutic use in psychosis. Drugs 33:31–49

Branchey M, Branchey L (1984) Patterns of psychotropic drug use and tardive dyskinesia. J Clin Psychopharmacol 4(1):41–45

Dahl SG (1986) Plasma level monitoring of antipsychotic drugs. Clinical utility. Clin Pharmacokinetics 11:36–61

Donlon PT, Tupin JP (1977) Successful suicides with thioridazine and mesoridazine. Arch Gen Psychiatry 34:955–957

Dupuis B, Catteau J, Dumon JP (1987) Comparison of propranolol, sotalol, and betaxolol in the treatment of neuroleptic-induced akathisia. Am J Psychiatry 144:802–805

Farde L, Wiesel FA, Halldin C, Sedvall G (1988) Central D2-dopamine receptor occupancy in schizophrenic patients treated with antipsychotic drugs. Arch Gen Psychiatry 45:71–76

Fowler NO, McCall, Chou TC, et al (1976) Electrocardiographic changes and cardiac arrhythmias in patients receiving psychotropic drugs. Am J Cardiology 37:223–230

Frichhione GL, Cassem NH, Hooberman D, Hobson D (1983) Intravenous lorazepam in neuroleptic-induced catatonia. J Clin Psychopharmacology 3:338–342

Friedman L, Weinrauch LA, D'Elia JA (1987) Metoclopramide-induced neuroleptic malignant syndrome. Arch Intern Med 147:1495–1497

Gardos G, Cole JO (1977) Weight reduction in schizophrenics by molindone. Am J Psychiatry 134:302–304

Guze BH, Baxter LR Jr (1985) Neuroleptic malignant syndrome. N Engl J Med 313:163–166

Hansen LB, Larsen NE (1985) Therapeutic advantages of monitoring plasma concentrations of perphenazine in clinical practice. Psychopharmacology 87:16–19

Herz M (1985) Prodromal symptoms and prevention of relapse in schizophrenia. J Clin Psychiatry 45 (11 Pt 2):22–25

Holley FO, Magliozzi JR, Stanski DR, et al (1983) Haloperidol kinetics after oral and intravenous doses. Clin Pharmacol Ther 33:477–484

Hollister LE (1970) Choice of anti-psychotic drugs. Am J Psychiatry 127:186–190

Hollister LE (1973) Clinical Use of Psychotherapeutic Drugs. Charles C Thomas, Springfield, IL

Hollister LE (1975) Hydroxyzine hydrochloride: Possible adverse cardiac interactions. Psychopharmacol Commun 1:61–65

Jain AK, Kewala S, Gershon S (1988) Antipsychotic drugs in schizophrenia: current issues. Int Clin Psychopharmacology 3:1–30

Jann MW, Ereshefsky L, Sklad SR, et al (1985) Effects of carbamazepine on plasma haloperidol levels. J Clin Psychopharmacol 5:106–109

Kane J, Honigfeld G, Singer J, Meltzer H (1988) Clozapine for the treatment-resistant schizophrenic. A double-blind comparison with chlorpromazine. Arch Gen Psychiatry 45(9):789–796

Karson CN, Weinberger DR, Bigelow L, Wyatt RJ (1982) Clonazepam treatment of chronic schizophrenia: negative results in a double-blind, placebo-controlled trial. Am J Psychiatr 139:1627–1628

Keck PE Jr, Pope HG Jr, McElroy S (1987) Frequency and presentation of neuroleptic malignant syndrome: a prospective study. Am J Psychiatry 144:1344–1346

Keepers G, Casey D (1987) Prediction of neuroleptic-induced dystonia. J Clin Psychopharmacol 7:342–345

Kim DY, Hollister LE (1984) Drug-refractory chronic schizophrenics: doses and plasma concentrations of thiothixene. J Clin Psychopharmacol 4:32–35

Kolakowska T, Williams AO, Ardern M, et al (1985) Schizophrenia with good and poor outcome. I. Early clinical features, response to neuroleptics and signs of organic dysfunction. Br J Psychiatry 146:229–246

Kovelman JA, Scheibel AB (1986) Biological substrates of schizophrenia. Acta Neurol Scand 73:1–22

Lathers CM, Lipka LJ (1987) Cardiac arrhythmia, sudden death and psychoactive agents. J Clin Pharmacol 27:1–14

Laursen AL, Gerlach J (1986) Antipsychotic effect of remoxipride, a new substituted benzamide with selective antidopamonergic activity. Acta Psychiatr Scand 73:17–21

Lehmann HE, Wilson WH, Deutsche M (1983) Minimal maintenance medication: effects of three dose schedules on relapse rates and symptoms in chronic schizophrenic outpatients. Compr Psychiatry 24:293–303

Magliozzi JR, Hollister LE, Arnold KV, Earle GM (1981) Relationship of serum haloperidol levels to clinical response in schizophrenic patients. Am J Psychiatry 138:365–367

Mandhanda R, Hirsch SR (1986) Does propranolol have an antipsychotic effect? A placebo-controlled study in acute schizophrenia. Br J Psychiatry 148:701–707

Marder SR, Van Putten T, Mintz J, et al (1984) Costs and benefits of two doses of fluphenazine. Arch Gen Psychiatry 41:1025–1029

Mavroidis ML, Kanter DR, Hirschowitz J, Garver DL (1983) Clinical response and haloperidol levels in schizophrenia. Psychopharmacology 81:354–356

Mavroidis ML, Kanter DR, Hirschowitz J, Garver DL (1984) Clinical relevance of thiothixene plasma levels. J Clin Psychopharmacol 4:133–137

McKenna PJ (1987) Pathology, phenomenology and the dopamine hypothesis of schizophrenia. Br J Psychiatry 151:288–301

Meredith TA, Aaberg TM, Willerson WD (1978) Progressive chorioretinopathy after receiving thioridazine. Arch Ophthalmol 96:1172–1176

Moore NC, Myendorff E, Yeragane V, et al (1987) Tiaspirone in schizophrenia. J Clin Psychopharmacol 7:98–101

Morgenstern H, Glazer WM, Gibowski LD, Holmberg S (1987) Predictors of tardive dyskinesia: results of a cross-sectional study in an outpatient population. J Chronic Dis 40:319–327

Myers JK, Weissman MM, Tischler GL, et al (1984) Six-month prevalence of psychiatric disorders in three communities. 1980 to 1983. Arch Gen Psychiatry 41:959–967

Niemegeers CJE, Janssen PAJ (1979) A systematic study of the pharmacological activities of dopamine antagonists. Life Sci 24:2201–2216

Overall JE, Hollister LE (1979) Comparative evaluation of research diagnostic criteria for schizophrenia. Arch Gen Psychiatry 36:1198–1205

Pugh CR, Steinist J, Priest RG (1983) Propranolol in schizophrenia: a double-blind placebo controlled trial of propranolol as adjunct to neuroleptic medication. Br J Psychiatr 143:151–155

Rivera-Calimlin L, Nasrullah H, Strauss J, Lasagna L (1976) Clinical response and plasma levels: effect of dose, dosage schedules and drug interactions on plasma chlorpromazine levels. Am J Psychiatry 133:646–652

Robins LN, Helzer JE, Weissman MM, et al (1984) Lifetime prevalence of specific psychiatric disorders in three sites. Arch Gen Psychiatry 41:949–958

Ross J, MacKenzie TB, Hanson DR, Charles CR (1987) Diltiazem for tardive dyskinesia (letter). Lancet 1:268

Salzman C, Green AI, Rodriguez-Villa F (1986) Benzodiazepines combined with neuroleptics for management of severe disruptive behavior. Psychosomatics 27:17–21

Schooler NR, Levine J, Severe JB, et al (1980) Prevention of relapse in schizophrenia. Arch Gen Psychiatry 37:16–24

Sherrington R, Brynjolfsson J, Petursson H, et al (1988) Localization of a susceptibility locus for schizophrenia on chromosome 5. Nature 336:164–170

Silver JM, Yudofsky SC, Kogan M, Katz BL (1986) Elevation of thioridazine plasma levels by propranolol. Am J Psychiatry 143:1290–1292

Simpson GM, Pi EH, Stramek JJ (1986) An update on tardive dyskinesia. Hos Community Psychiatry 37:362–369

Small J, Milstein V, Marhenke JD, et al (1987) Treatment outcome with clozapine in tardive dyskinesia, neuroleptic sensitivity, and treatment-resistant psychosis. J Clin Psychiatry 48:263–267

Smith WO, Clark ML (1980) Self-induced water intoxication in schizophrenic patients. Am J Psychiatry 137:1055–1060

Stahl SM (1986) Tardive dyskinesia: natural history studies assist the pursuit of preventive therapies. Psychol Med 16:491–494

Stevens JR (1988) Is there a neuropathology of schizophrenia? Biol Psychiatry 24:123–128

Van Putten T, Marder SR, May PRA, et al (1985) Plasma levels of haloperidol and clinical response. Psychopharmacol Bull 21:69–72

Vincent FM (1980) Phenothiazine-induced phenytoin intoxication. Ann Intern Med 93:56–57

Weiden P, Mann JJ, Haas G, (1987) Clinical nonrecognition of neuroleptic-induced movement disorders: a cautionary tale. Am J Psychiatry 144:1148–1153

Zohar J, Shemesh Z, Belmaker RH (1986) Utility of neuroleptic blood levels in the treatment of acute psychosis. J Clin Psychiatry 47:600–603

# 6

---

# MOOD-STABILIZING DRUGS

## HISTORY

Treatment of manic-depressive illness in the not-too-distant past was unsatisfactory. Before the advent of antipsychotic drugs, reliance was placed primarily on electroconvulsive therapy (ECT) or, in a few places, on atropine coma. Various sedatives, such as barbiturates or bromides, were used to provide brief respites from the most severe symptoms of this disorder, but with no lasting or specific benefit. Thus, patients were often hospitalized for very long periods, and fatalities were not unusual. Although today fatalities from manic-depressive illness are likely to be suicide, such deaths accounted for only 1.3 percent of those occurring in the Brooklyn State Hospital from 1927 to 1932; 40 percent of the deaths were due to simple "exhaustion" (Derby, 1933).

The advent of antipsychotic drugs in the 1950s made it possible to mitigate the course of manic-depressive illness. Chlorpromazine and reserpine were effective in reducing the marked agitation and elevation of mood seen in mania, but their side effects counterbalanced these benefits. Patients complained of being heavily drugged, which was usually the case. Sometimes these drugs precipitated a serious depressive episode in a patient who was previously manic. Nonetheless, control of the most severe symptoms of manic-depressive illness was much better than before. Quite possibly this development delayed the acceptance of lithium as a treatment of mania.

Lithium had been introduced into medicine by Garrod in 1859 as a treatment for gout. Lithium bromide was one of the most frequently used bromide salts, which were used by Hammond not only to treat epilepsy but also mania and melancholia (Amdisen, 1987). However, the lithium ion itself attracted little attention until the late 1940s. At that time, patients in congestive heart failure were usually put on salt-restricted diets as well as organic mercurial diuretics, and lithium chloride, which tasted like sodium chloride, was used as a salt substitute. In retrospect, one can hardly imagine a better set of circumstances for producing lethal lithium toxicity, which is exactly what happened. After several

127

deaths were reported in 1949, lithium itself was considered too dangerous for any type of medical treatment.

That same year, in Australia, John Cade was looking for toxic substances in the urine of manic patients and found that such urine could kill rodents, probably due to the presence of urea. In trying to determine how uric acid might modify the toxicity of urea, he selected lithium urate, the most soluble salt, and administered it to his animals. Somewhat surprisingly, lithium urate had a calming action in these animals, as did lithium carbonate. He reasoned that in some fashion, lithium ion protected against the toxicity of urine from manic patients. Cade then decided to administer lithium carbonate to manic patients, and an amazingly fortuitous choice of dose, 600 mg three times daily, proved optimal. Responses in all 10 manic patients treated with lithium were gratifying (Cade, 1970).

Further studies of other ions in the alkali metal series were initiated, and the clinical import of the discovery was all but lost. In Denmark, Schou continued to explore the clinical use of lithium, repeatedly confirming its efficacy for managing acute mania and ultimately its efficacy for preventing the recurrent attacks of the illness, which contribute so much to morbidity (Schou, 1957). He confirmed the narrow range of clinical doses and serum concentrations. By the mid-1960s, lithium had become recognized throughout most of the world as a treatment for manic-depressive disorder. It did not become available in the United States until 1970, one of the many examples of the "drug lag" operating here.

In 1971, the most recent of developments occurred. Until then, lithium was completely unique in its multiplicity of effects on manic-depressive illness. Then it was discovered in Japan that carbamazepine, an anticonvulsant, had a similar spectrum of effects. Once the first article in English was published in 1973, further confirmation came over the next several years. This discovery has greatly broadened the scope of research on manic-depressive illness and led to the search for other compounds, mainly anticonvulsants, with mood-stabilizing effects.

## NATURE OF MANIC-DEPRESSIVE ILLNESS
### Nosologic Development

In the nineteenth century, the terms *manic-depressive illness* and *manic-depressive psychosis* were coined to describe an illness characterized by unpredictable alternations of extreme mood states—mania and depression. This illness was distinguished from schizophrenia by its relative lack of unrelenting deterioration. However, since the publication of the third edition of the *Diagnostic and Statistical Manual for Mental Disorders* in 1980 (DSM-III), the term *bipolar disorder* has been substituted for these earlier terms. In the current revised third edition of the DSM (DSM-IIIR), three forms of bipolar disorder can be diagnosed: manic, depressed, or mixed.

The term *bipolar disorder* carries with it an implicit assumption about the relationship between the prevalent mood states that may or may not be justified. The implication is that these mood states exist on opposite poles of a continuum with normal mood in the middle. However, alternative relationships between mania and depression are also possible (Fig. 6-1). Certainly patients pass from mania into depression and back again frequently, but it is far from clear that they always go through periods of normal mood to do so. The fact that depression often follows mania immediately and vice versa, and the occasional simultaneous presence of mania and depression in the same patient, seems to contradict this model. Furthermore, this terminology may lead one to assume that there are fundamental similarities between bipolar depression and unipolar depression, which remains controversial.

Nonetheless, the natural history of manic-depressive illness has been well described. This illness most frequently begins in the third decade of life, but rarely after age 50. In contrast, unipolar depressions may occur for the first time over a wide time span, with a median age of onset of 43 years. Almost all patients with either manic-depressive illness or unipolar depression will have recurrent episodes. Cycle length is dependent on age of onset, number of episodes (usually shorter cycles with more episodes), and duration of the previous cycle. Both illnesses are long lasting, so that prophylactic treatment may be required for at least a decade (Angst and Grof, 1976).

Only a few years ago, manic-depressive illness was considered to be rather uncommon, but it is now a frequently diagnosed, serious emotional disorder. An older literature suggested that many patients diagnosed as manic-depressives ultimately became recognized as having an agitated form of paranoid schizophrenia (grandiosity, bellicosity, paranoid thoughts, and overactivity). This conclusion, whether or not it was justified, prevailed, for the latter diagnosis became common and the former rare. Now the pendulum has swung almost 180

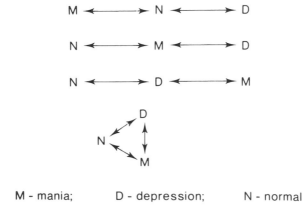

M - mania;      D - depression;      N - normal

**Fig. 6-1.** Alternatives to the bipolar model of manic-depressive disorder. The classic bipolar model is shown at the top, with mania and depression at the poles of the continuum and a normal mood in between. Other possible relationships are shown. M, mania; D, depression; N, normal.

degrees. Of 50 patients admitted with a diagnosis of mania, 28 were found to have been previously diagnosed as schizophrenic. Irritability was more prominent than euphoria. A high preponderance of psychotic symptoms may have led to the misdiagnosis. In fact, it is now well known that psychotic symptoms, even those characterized as Schneiderian first-rank in nature, are common in extreme forms of mania or depression.

Despite this trend toward an increase in the diagnosis of the disorder, it has been estimated that as many as one-third to one-half of patients with manic depressive illness are not receiving treatment and that 20 percent of those being treated for it do not have it. Thus, many cases are still misdiagnosed.

# Differential Diagnosis

During the acute episode, the depressed phase of manic-depressive illness is indistinguishable from that of unipolar depression. Therefore, the presence of mania is critical for diagnosing manic-depressive illness. Mania is characterized by a predominantly elevated, expansive or irritable mood; this mood change is obligatory for the diagnosis. It must have lasted for at least 1 week or have had consequences severe enough to lead to hospitalization. In addition, according to DSM-IIIR criteria, at least three (or four, if the mood is irritable) of the following symptoms must also be present: (1) inflated self-esteem or grandiosity; (2) decreased need for sleep; (3) more talkative than usual; (4) flight of ideas or racing thoughts; (5) distractibility; (6) an increase in activity; (7) foolish but pleasurable behavior. A single documented instance of mania, even so-called secondary mania induced by the administration of tricyclic or MAO inhibitor antidepressants, should be adequate to make the diagnosis of manic-depressive illness. Mania induced by antidepressants has been termed bipolar 3, as contrasted with bipolar 1 (in which mania accompanies depression) and bipolar 2 (in which hypomania accompanies depression). Such subclassification has not added much to understanding.

## Schizophrenia

As has been mentioned, confusion between schizophrenia and manic-depressive disorder is common, for, as with most pyschiatric disorders, a number of nonspecific manifestations are shared. In particular, the paranoid and disorganized (hebephrenic) forms of schizophrenia can resemble mania. A major distinguishing feature of schizophrenia is the presence of a formal thought disorder, emotional blunting, and other negative symptoms.

## Schizoaffective Disorders

Patients with schizoaffective disorders are still difficult to classify. One possibility is that such patients have a biologic predisposition both to schizophrenia and to a mood disorder. Another is that the cause of some forms of schizophrenia and mood disorders are very closely linked. Attempts to use discriminant analytic techniques to separate these two entities based on variables concerned with the course of illness and ratings of psychopathology over long periods of time have met with only limited success (Brockington et al., 1979). Lateral ventricular enlargement has been found in patients with both schizophrenia and manic-depressive illness (Rieder et al., 1983). Finally, schizophrenia and bipolar mood disorder are both found at relatively high rates in the families of patients with schizoaffective disorder (Gershon et al., 1988). After all, the boundary between at least some forms of these two disorders may be more apparent than real.

## Personality Disorders

Several personality disorders recognized by DSM IIIR are characterized by an instability of mood. These include antisocial personality disorder, borderline personality disorder, histrionic personality disorder, and narcissistic personality disorder. Cyclothymic personality disorder, as defined by DSM-II, is now known simply as cyclothymia in DSM-IIIR and is included in the mood disorders. For practical purposes, it may be considered a minor variant of bipolar disorders.

In all these disorders, the alternations of mood are of a lesser degree than in manic-depressive illness and are more often tied to an interpersonal or psychological insult. Yet the boundaries among these disorders and between them and manic-depressive illness remain to be validated by biologic studies. It is also relevant to note that some investigators have claimed that both lithium and carbamazepine are effective for the management of these disorders as well.

## Attention Deficit Disorder

Attention deficit disorder with hyperactivity may be very difficult to distinguish from mania in children. Children cannot always articulate fine shades of mood, and the outward behaviors of these two syndromes can be identical. However, attempts at treatment usually bring such mistakes to light. Administration of stimulants to children with mania can cause a dramatic worsening of symptoms.

# Etiology and Pathogenesis

A growing consensus supports a genetic basis for manic-depressive illness, although results are still controversial. Evidence for a linkage between illness and the F9 locus for coagulation factor IX was found in 10 of 24 families of manic-depressive patients with two or more affected relatives (Mendlewicz, 1987). Earlier, the gene for the illness had been linked to genes for color blindness and glucose-6-phosphate dehydrogenase deficiency, both of which are located on the X-chromosome (Baron et al., 1987). A study of Amish communities in the United States revealed a family with 14 of 81 members with manic-depressive illness. Two markers were found for a gene on chromosome 11 that predisposes those with the gene to develop the illness. Although the gene is inherited in an autosomal dominant pattern, penetrance was incomplete, as only 60 to 80 percent of those who inherit the gene develop the illness (Egeland,

1987). Two other groups, one working with families in Iceland, the other with patients in North America, have found no genetic markers (Hodgkinson et al., 1987). Thus, the matter remains unsettled; the illness is likely to be heterogeneous.

Whether hereditary predisposition alone can explain the expression of manic-depressive illness remains open to question. One is tempted to believe that episodes of the disorder follow some life stress, yet such associations are not made easily. One may still wish to consider an interactive model in which heredity sets the stage for the disorder and life stresses provide the cues for its clinical appearance.

The neurochemical mechanism for the expression of manic-depressive symptoms remains unknown. As the depressive phase of manic-depressive illness is phenomenologically identical to unipolar depression, pathogenetic models of unipolar depression may apply to this illness as well (see Chapter 4). Several neurotransmitter systems have been implicated in the pathogenesis of mania, including norepinephrine, serotonin, and dopamine. Increases in norepinephrine and serotonin activity have been linked to mania by virtue of the fact that tricyclic antidepressants, which block the reuptake of these two biogenic amines, can induce manic episodes in bipolar patients when they are treated for depression (Wehr and Goodwin, 1987). Dopamine can be implicated in mania because of the fact that neuroleptics are effective in the treatment of mania, even those such as pimozide that are highly specific as dopamine D-2 antagonists (Post et al., 1980).

A cholinergic–noradrenergic balance hypothesis of manic-depressive illness was proposed in the early 1970s (Janowsky et al., 1972). Bipolar depression could be explained as a relative predominance of acetylcholine over norepinephrine activity, whereas mania was a relative predominance of norepinephrine over acetylcholine activity. Three types of circadian rhythm abnormalities have been described: blunting of amplitudes, advanced phases, and doubling of the normal sleep–wake cycle to 48 hours (Wehr et al., 1983). Whether these changes are the result or a cause of the disorder is unclear.

# PHARMACOLOGY OF LITHIUM
## Pharmacokinetics

Absorption of lithium is rapid following an oral dose and is virtually complete within 6 to 8 hours. The type of lithium salt used is inconsequential for absorption. Peak plasma levels occur within 30 minutes to 2 hours after the dose. Plasma concentrations of lithium in patients on a three-times-daily dose schedule may vary over a twofold range, rising as each dose is absorbed and then falling during the long period in which doses are not given. Clinical monitoring of plasma levels uses those obtained at the nadir (Thornhill, 1981).

Lithium is distributed in the total body water, shifting slowly into cells. Distinct two-compartment characteristics are evident. The slow entry into cells may account for the delay of several days before full clinical responses are noted.

Exit from cells is likewise slow, which probably accounts for the slow clearing of confusion and other signs of toxicity after an overdose. Various tissues concentrate lithium to various degrees. No protein binding occurs. Lithium levels in the cerebrospinal fluid peak 24-hours later than those in the extracellular fluid and generally reach a concentration only 50 percent of that in plasma. Passage into the brain is slow, but some areas contain levels higher than those in plasma. Apparent volumes of distribution under steady-state conditions have ranged from 50 to 90 percent of body weight, somewhat higher than the actual body content of water, which is 50 to 55 percent (Nielsen-Kudsk and Amdisen, 1979).

Lithium is 95 percent excreted in the urine. Although it passes freely through the glomerulus, only 20 percent of filtered lithium is excreted as it is reabsorbed in the proximal tubule. Clearance rates have varied from 7 to 38 mg/min, about 20 percent of the creatinine clearance. The elimination half-life in normal persons given single doses varies between 12 and 21 hours; after long-term administration the half-life tends to increase (Goodnick et al., 1981). Whether or not manics retain abnormal amounts of lithium is still uncertain.

Lithium clearance is reduced by thiazide diuretics. In the case of chlorothiazide, a 500-mg daily dose reduces clearance by 40 percent and a dose of 1000 mg reduces clearance by 68 percent. Thus, doses of lithium should be adjusted during concomitant treatment with thiazides (Himmelhoch et al., 1977).

Lithium is also excreted in saliva, and within individuals the ratio of plasma concentration to salivary concentration is fixed. Once this ratio has been established, saliva rather than blood can suffice for monitoring lithium concentrations (Groth et al., 1974). However, most clinicians probably prefer to collect blood from adults rather than take the time and effort to collect saliva; the latter may be preferable for monitoring levels in children.

Of all the psychotherapeutic drugs for which plasma or serum determinations are available, lithium is without doubt the one for which monitoring of levels is mandatory. One can scarcely conceive of using this drug, with such a small therapeutic margin, without the ability to monitor serum concentrations. The range of therapeutic concentrations is 0.6 to 1.4 mEq/L, whereas those effective for maintenance treatment are from 0.4 to 0.9 mEq/L. These are nadir values; that is, they are measured on blood samples taken 12 hours following the last dose, when all absorption and accumulation of lithium from daily dosing has ceased. Steady-state plasma concentrations are generally attained after about 5 days of treatment, assuming the elimination half-life with chronic dosing to be approximately 24 hours.

Serum lithium concentrations may not always correlate directly with intraneuronal concentrations. The latter may be altered by circumstances other than the serum lithium concentrations. Whether erythrocyte lithium concentrations are a better guide than serum has never been settled. The ratios of lithium in erythrocytes to serum seem to be higher in manic patients, and patients with high ratios seem to respond better to lithium (Swann et al., 1987). In any case, the values reported from the laboratory cannot be slavishly followed but should be used only as a guide. Many instances of clinical toxicity occur with serum concentrations thought to be in the therapeutic range, and conversely, lithium can be therapeutically effective at "subtherapeutic" levels, especially in the elderly (Jefferson and Greist, 1981). A summary of the kinetic parameters of lithium is given in Table 6-1.

## Mechanisms of Action

One can safely say that almost 40 years of investigation have failed to establish the essential pharmacologic actions of lithium. The many actions that have been discovered were recently reviewed (Wood and Goodwin, 1987). The possibility that lithium might substitute for one or more important electrolytes, namely $Na^+$, $K^+$, $Ca^{++}$, and $Mg^{++}$, and that such actions might be related to its therapeutic effects seems obvious. Lithium substitutes most readily for $Na^+$, owing in part to its similar ionic radius, and therefore could alter a variety of processes linked to the functioning of the $Na^+/K^+$–ATPase. However, it is well known to inhibit a variety of $Ca^{++}$-dependent biochemical processes as well. Lithium, along with $Ca^{++}$ and $Mg^{++}$, would also act directly to stabilize cell membranes, thus having nonspecific biophysical effects on neuronal function. The role of $Ca^{++}$ may be crucial, as neural mechanisms hypothesized to explain various psychopharmacologic treatments of bipolar illness are controlled by $Ca^{++}$ (Meltzer, 1986).

It might be more reasonable to investigate lithium's mechanism(s) of action by examining its effects on the neurotransmitter systems hypothesized to be involved in mood disorders. Of these systems, the effects of lithium on serotonin function have been studied in the greatest depth. Lithium has both presynaptic and postsynaptic effects on serotonin function. In one animal study, long-term administration of lithium was shown to increase $K^+$-stimulated release of serotonin and decrease postsynaptic serotonin 5-$HT_2$ receptor binding from the hippocampus but not cortex (Treiser et al., 1981). Although these two effects appear to be opposite, the overall action of lithium on the serotonin system could be claimed to be "stabilizing." Moreover, these effects may be similar to the effects of tricyclic antidepressants, which can also down-regulate serotonin 5-$HT_2$ receptors. Thus, one hypothesis, based on a number of circumstantial arguments, is that lithium acts through serotonin (Muller-Oerlinghausen, 1985).

**Table 6-1. Pharmacokinetic Parameters of Lithium**

| | |
|---|---|
| Bioavailability | Complete and rapid absorption in 6–8 hours |
| Protein-binding | None |
| Volume of distribution | 50–90 percent of body weight; possible sequestration in bone |
| Plasma half-life | 20 hours |
| Metabolites | None |
| Excretion | Virtually all through kidney; lithium clearance is 0.2 creatinine clearance |
| Therapeutic plasma concentration | 0.6–1.4 mEq/L; 0.6–1.0 mEq/L maintenance |

One of the earliest studies of lithium's neurochemical effects indicated that it could increase the terminal reuptake of norepinephrine (Colburn et al., 1967). However, this effect may not persist with long-term administration (Cameron and Smith, 1980). In animals, lithium has also been shown to block the ability of neuroleptics to cause an upregulation of dopamine D-2 receptors. This finding may have some pertinence regarding the prophylactic effects of lithium against mania and may also suggest a role for lithium in preventing neuroleptic-induced movement disorders.

One of the most interesting recent findings involves the effect of lithium on a newly discovered second-messenger system, the phosphatidylinositol cycle. The elements of this intraneuronal signaling system are found in Figure 6-2.

An alternation of phosphorylation and dephosphorylation reactions yields two second-messenger molecules, diacylglycerol and inositol triphosphate. Lithium interferes with this cycle by blocking the conversion of inositol monophosphate to inositol by inositol monophosphate phosphatase (Sherman et al., 1981). However, the physiologic consequences for neurotransmitter receptor systems linked to this second-messenger system remain under investigation. In one study, lithium pretreatment produced a dampening effect (Menkes et al., 1986). It is of great interest that the muscarinic acetylcholine receptor is among those neurotransmitter receptors linked to the phosphatidylinositol second-messenger system in the brain. Given the cholinergic–adrenergic balance hypothesis of manic-depressive illness mentioned earlier, this suggests that the antimanic actions of lithium might be attributed to its effects on acetylcholine through this second-messenger system.

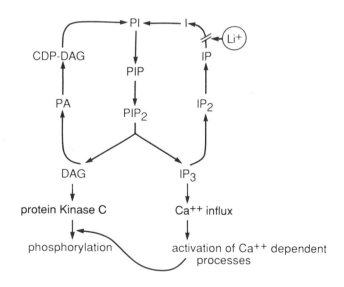

**Fig. 6-2.** The Phosphatidylinositol Second Messenger System. PIP$_2$, phosphatidylinositol bisphosphate; PI, phosphatidylinositol; PA, phosphatidate; CDP-DAG, cytidine diphosphodiacylglycerol; PIP, phosphatidylinositol phosphate; IP, inositol monophosphate; IP$_2$, inositol bisphosphate; IP$_3$, inositol trisphosphate. (Modified from Snider et al. (1987), with permission.)

# CLINICAL USE OF LITHIUM
## Preliminary Workup

Before starting treatment, one should obtain laboratory tests that might include a complete blood count, urinalysis, the common battery of plasma chemistry assays, and a panel of thyroid function tests. The urinalysis may provide evidence of acute or chronic renal disease, although the values for serum creatinine and electrolytes from the biochemical battery might be more pertinent. The thyroid tests would be measured primarily as benchmarks for future testing of possible antithyroid actions of lithium. If any questions of renal disease arise, a creatinine clearance test is advisable; the presence of renal disease that either impairs function or makes it variable might be considered a contraindication. Older patients might do well to have a baseline ECG recording. Severe cardiac disease requiring the use of diuretics might also be a contraindication. Women in the child-bearing years should be assessed for pregnancy before treatment.

## Doses

By far, the most common form of lithium is lithium carbonate. It is now available in slow-release 450-mg dosage forms, as well as conventional 300-mg capsules. If one requires a liquid preparation, lithium citrate is available.

One should consider the patient's body weight and age in selecting the appropriate starting dose of lithium carbonate. The initial volume of distribution of lithium will be the body water, which is approximately 50 percent of body weight for adult women and 55 percent for adult men. The proportion of body water may decrease slightly at older age levels, as will renal function. Any patient past age 50 is likely to have decreased creatinine clearance, which may drop to 50 percent or less of normal values without apparent elevation of serum creatinine. Thus, large patients may require larger doses, but older patients will generally require a dose less than that predicted for their size.

One method of determining the lithium carbonate dose is to administer a single test dose of 600 mg and then measure the serum concentration 24 hours later. According to the level at that time, one can make a prediction about the daily dose needed to provide serum concentrations between 0.6 and 1.2 mEq/L (Cooper et al., 1973). This procedure may be of particular use in patients with mild renal impairment or any other condition that might lead to unpredictable lithium serum concentrations. This procedure has been modified with a change to a 900-mg test dose and formulation of a new nomogram for predicting daily dose based on serum lithium levels at 24 hours (Rosenberg et al., 1987).

A direct calculation of dose based on body weight will also predict therapeutic levels of lithium measured after 7 days of treatment. High (0.72 mEq/kg/day) and medium (0.5 mEq/kg/day) doses were more effective than a low (0.24 mEq/kg/day) dose. In fact, the lowest dose was no better than placebo. Serum lithium concentrations after 7 days of treatment averaged 1.06, 0.91, and 0.43 mEq/L, respectively (Stokes et al., 1976). The medium dose might be one worth considering as a starting dose for most patients, although the fixed unit sizes of conventional lithium carbonate preparations (300 mg or 8 mEq) may prohibit giving the exact calculated amount.

## Monitoring Serum Lithium Concentrations

One should attain an initial therapeutic plasma concentration between 0.6 and 1.4 mEq/L. Levels less than these may not be fully effective, and nothing seems to be gained by exceeding the upper limit (Schou, 1988). Usual doses range from 600 mg to 1200 mg daily, and should be guided by serum concentrations. For instance, if the patient received 600 mg daily and had a plasma concentration of 0.5 mEq/L, a dose adjustment to 900 mg daily (an increase of 50 percent) could be expected to yield an approximate serum concentration of 0.7 to 0.8 mEq/L. Doses should be carefully titrated to the needs of patients. It should be adequate to measure serum levels of lithium weekly during the first 4 weeks of treatment and less often (every 4 to 6 weeks) thereafter. The trend toward lower doses and lower serum concentrations may reduce side effects or complications of treatment. However, patients who do not respond should be treated with the highest doses that are tolerable. Table 6-2 summarizes a practical approach to selecting an initial lithium dosage, and modifying it based upon serum lithium concentrations.

## Dosage Schedules

The long half-life of lithium makes single daily dose administration of drug possible, but large single doses may not be well tolerated because of gastric irritation. Most often, the dose is divided equally during the day into two to six doses. Frequent doses can alleviate some gastrointestinal symptoms. In lieu of frequent doses, one might try a sustained-release preparation of lithium carbonate. Medication taken with or shortly after meals is less likely to cause gastrointestinal distress, which can be confused with toxicity.

### Table 6-2. Approach to Determination of Lithium Dose

| | |
|---|---|
| Initial dose | 0.5 mEq/kg |
| *Example:* | 80 kg man = 40 mEq |
| | 8 mEq/300 mg dose unit |
| | $\dfrac{40}{8}$ = 5 dose units, or approximately 1500 mg |

Obtain plasma concentration after 7 days
> *Example:*   Reported concentration is 0.9 mEq/L; clinical response is inadequate; there are no signs of toxicity

To increase plasma concentration to 1.2 mEq/L, increase dose by 1/3, to 2100 mg (approximate)

To reduce plasma concentration for prophylaxis to 0.6 mEq/L, decrease dose to 50 percent

## Evaluating the Response to Lithium

One should expect a lag period of several days even after therapeutic serum levels have been attained for the antimanic effect of lithium to be clearly apparent. The overall success rate for the manic phase of manic-depressive illness is estimated to be 60 to 80 percent. This means that a sizable group of patients will be lithium resistant, which may provide support for the notion that manic-depressive illness is heterogeneous, occurring through several pathogenetic mechanisms. Fortunately, many alternative treatments can be tried for patients unresponsive to lithium.

No single factor, beyond attaining adequate serum lithium levels, has an absolute predictive value for the outcome of lithium treatment. In general, the more secure the diagnosis of manic-depressive illness, the more favorable the response. A cyclothymic premorbid personality, a pyknic body build, and a family history of manic-depressive disorder may augur for a positive response. Nonresponders are likely to be those who have previously failed lithium treatment, those with frequently cycling attacks (four or more a year for 2 to 3 years preceding treatment), those with previous history of schizophrenia or schizoaffective symptoms, and those with chronic anxiety and obsessive features (Petursson, 1979).

## Prophylactic Treatment of Manic-Depressive Illness

The natural history of manic-depressive illness is such that once the diagnosis has been made, it is likely that the patient will have a subsequent course marked by multiple recurrences of major manic or depressive episodes. Even patients who have not had a full-blown manic episode, but who have had hypomania as well as depression, have a high risk for recurrence. Both major manic or major depressive episodes can be highly disruptive and lead to suicide. Therefore, one is obliged to consider prophylactic treatment for all patients.

In 14 studies of bipolar illness, lithium maintenance was found to decrease the number of recurrences by 50 percent as compared with placebo. Patients with previously established rapid-cycling (three or more episodes a year) responded less well. Therefore, continuation treatment with lithium is well established, though by no means perfect. Even an early recurrence during prophylactic treatment should not lead to its abandonment, as the preventive effect may take several months to develop (Consensus Development Conference, 1984).

Breakthroughs of either mania or depression should first lead to a check of serum lithium levels, which may be too low owing to noncompliance. Thyroid function might be checked, as lithium-induced hypothyroidism may aggravate mood disorders. The addition of an antipsychotic for mania or an antidepressant for depression may be required. Tricyclic antidepressants are thought to instigate rapid-cycling in some patients (Wehr and Goodwin, 1987); MAO inhibitors or the second generation antidepressants may be a better choice.

Doses of lithium to be used during maintenance treatment should be relatively low, with associated serum levels near 0.6 mEq/L. Such conservatism reduces both morbidity and side effects during prophylaxis (Coppen et al., 1983). Failure to maintain a patient in remission on lithium may call for either the addition or substitution of carbamazepine. Among 90 bipolar patients treated with pro-phylactic lithium, 48 percent responded to lithium as the sole mood-stabilizing drug. Thirty-four lithium nonresponders were then treated with the addition of carbamazepine, which caused response in 5, or the substitution of the drug, which caused 17 more to respond (Fawcett and Kravitz, 1985).

Sudden cessation of lithium during prophylactic treatment should be avoided. Seven of 14 patients switched to placebo in a blind controlled trial had relapse and two additional patients had incipient relapse. Relapses started 13 to 19 days after placebo substitution (Mander and Loudon, 1988).

## Other Indications for Lithium

Schizoaffective disorder is characterized by a mixture of schizophrenic symptoms and extreme mood states, either in the form of depression or manic excitement. These episodes are difficult to distinguish from psychotic unipolar depressions or episodes of true mania. A comparison of chlorpromazine and lithium in 83 patients so diagnosed proved that chlorpromazine was more effective for highly excited patients with no difference in more mildly active patients (Prien et al., 1972). Thus, it is likely that in schizoaffective disorder, concurrent lithium and neuroleptic treatment may be superior to antipsychotic drugs alone (Biederman et al., 1979). Lithium alone is rarely sufficient.

Lithium cannot be regarded as a primary treatment for schizophrenia. However, lithium, either alone or when added to an ongoing neuroleptic, may be partially effective, even in alleviating the fundamental psychotic symptoms of the disease. Schizophrenic patients who are lithium-responsive tend to have shorter durations of illness (Hirschowitz et al., 1980). One should also consider the possibility that diagnostic difficulties in distinguishing paranoid schizo-phrenia from manic-depressive illness could lead one to think that a schizophre-nic has responded to lithium when the proper diagnosis should have been manic-depressive illness.

Psychotically depressed patients who had not responded to a combination of antidepressant–antipsychotic medication were treated with the addition of lithium. Lithium was effective in 8 of 9 patients with bipolar depression but in only 3 of 12 with unipolar depression; electroconvulsive treatment (ECT) was effective in 9 of 15 other unipolar depressed patients (Nelson, 1986). The value of lithium as a treatment for unipolar depression has never really been well established.

Alcoholism often appears to be associated with depression and mania. However, this association appears to derive in part from the fact that alcoholic intoxication can resemble manic excitement and the dysphoria encountered during early abstinence from alcohol can resemble depression. Furthermore, patients with manic-depressive illness often self-medicate with alcohol. There appears to be little or no genetic association between alcoholism and manic-depressive illness (Schuckit, 1986).

Lithium was tried several years ago as a treatment for chronic alcoholism. The end point, of disabling drinking episodes, was a bit vague, but statistical analysis proved lithium to be more effective than placebo (Kline et al., 1974). A recent study of 104 alcoholics in a blind, placebo-controlled trial of lithium who were followed for 12 months indicated virtually no response for noncompliant patients; 31 to 44 percent of partially compliant patients, who did not attain therapeutic serum lithium levels, became abstinent; 67 percent of patients who were fully compliant, with therapeutic concentrations of lithium, became abstinent (Fawcett et al., 1987). Thus, it appears that something good may happen.

Episodes of uncontrollable aggressive behavior have been considered as a potential indication for lithium. Evidence to support such use is not overwhelming. Hyperactivity associated with mental retardation is often exceedingly difficult to treat. During a 4-month blind cross-over trial comparing lithium with placebo in 42 mentally handicapped persons, 73 percent of patients on lithium showed a reduction in aggression during treatment, with a significant difference between the lithium and placebo groups. Side effects were of little consequence (Craft et al., 1987). It is difficult to predict how long these beneficial effects might last.

# Drug Interactions

## Pharmacokinetic

Renal clearance of lithium is decreased by thiazide diuretics but may be increased by water diuretics, such as aminophylline. Loop diuretics, such as furosemide, have little effect. Depletion of sodium, for whatever reason, favors retention of lithium.

Prostaglandin synthetase inhibitors, such as phenylbutazone, indomethacin, diclofenac, and probably a number of other nonsteroidal antiinflammatory drugs, decrease renal clearance of lithium and increase serum levels (Reimann and Frohlich, 1981). This action is related to inhibition of renal prostaglandins. Fortunately, no such interactions have yet been described for the most commonly used analgesics, aspirin and acetaminophen.

## Pharmacodynamic

The interaction described with haloperidol has diminished in importance with the passage of time. There seems to be little doubt that lithium given concurrently with any of the neuroleptics can increase their neurotoxicity. Delirium, seizures, encephalopathy, and grossly abnormal EEGs were encountered in four patients in whom lithium was added to thioridazine (Spring, 1979). However, the combination of lithium and neuroleptics may be indicated in some manic-depressive and schizoaffective patients. A good rule of thumb is to avoid high neuroleptic doses and serum lithium levels above 1.0 mEq/L when using the combination.

# ADVERSE EFFECTS

The side effects associated with lithium treatment occur at varying times after treatment. Some are harmless, whereas others may augur the onset of toxicity (Simard et al., 1989). It is important to distinguish which side effects may herald toxicity. Table 6-3 shows the distinction that might be made.

## General

A survey of lithium side effects in 237 patients on long-term treatment found only 10 percent of patients without any complaints. Two-thirds of the patients had one or two complaints, and one-fourth had three or more. About one-half complained of hand tremors, two-thirds of increased thirst, one-fifth of diarrhea, and one-fifth of weight gain, and one-tenth of edema of face or legs (Vestergaard et al., 1980).

## Central Nervous System

A fine, rapid tremor is an early side effect. Propranolol has been used successfully to treat it; metoprolol is a possible alternative. Fatigue, lassitude, muscle weakness, and subtle cogwheel rigidity may occur, as do more evident extrapyramidal symptoms. These are not responsive to antiparkinsonism drugs and appear late in treatment, unlike the extrapyramidal syndromes from

**Table 6-3.** Frequent Side Effects and Signs of Lithium Toxicity

|  | Side Effects | | Toxicity |
|---|---|---|---|
|  | Early | Late | Impending |
| Gastrointestinal |  |  |  |
| Nausea, loose stools | + |  |  |
| Vomiting, diarrhea |  |  | + |
| Neuromuscular |  |  |  |
| Fine tremor, hands | + | + |  |
| Coarse tremor, hands |  |  | + |
| Sleepiness |  |  | + |
| Vertigo |  |  | + |
| Dysarthria |  |  | + |
| Metabolic–Endocrine |  |  |  |
| Polyuria | + | + |  |
| Edema |  | + |  |
| Weight gain |  | + |  |
| Goiter, hypothyroidism |  | + |  |

antipsychotic drugs (Tyrer et al., 1980). Cognitive effects may be difficult to identify, the patient merely appearing to be apathetic.

More severe symptoms and signs can occur, such as dysarthria, ataxia, apasia, muscle twitching, and hyperreflexia. These constitute definite evidence of toxicity and mandate a decrease in lithium dose, regardless of the serum levels.

## Renal

An extensive literature has developed concerning the chronic renal effects of lithium, especially after the report of interstitial nephritis during long-term lithium therapy (Hestbech et al., 1977). The prevalence of these changes in humans is still undetermined. About 25 percent of patients in long-term treatment are found to have a nephropathy characterized by a reduction in concentrating ability. This reduction is not related to the degree of polyuria and takes about 7 years to develop, with a minimum of 3 years. The degree of damage to the renal interstitium was dependent on serum lithium concentration and duration of treatment (Albrecht et al., 1980). However, another study has suggested that manic patients, even those who have never received lithium, have a lower than normal ability to concentrate urine, which is further reduced by lithium treatment (Wahlin et al., 1980). Decreases in creatinine clearance during long-term lithium treatment seem to be rare. Lithium clearance was measured in 44 patients treated for an average of 8 years. The average renal clearance was 21.6 ml/min; the clearance in 26 affective disorder patients never treated with lithium was the same (Helmar and Rafaelsen, 1987). Although serum creatinine is notorious for correlating poorly with creatinine clearance, serum beta-2-microglobulin may correlate better. It remains to be seen whether this measure will detect more instances of decreased creatinine clearance (Samiy and Rosnick, 1987).

Polydipsia and polyuria are common early side effects of lithium treatment, occurring at therapeutic plasma concentrations. They are not a manifestation of toxicity. The principal physiologic mechanism involved is the loss of the ability of the distal tubule to conserve water under the influence of antidiuretic hormone (ADH, vasopressin). Excessive free-water clearance causes the increased fluid intake.

Resistance of such lithium-induced nephrogenic diabetes insipidus to vasopressin has led to other attempts at therapy. Amiloride blunts the inhibitory effect of lithium on water transport in the renal collecting tubule. Its clinical use in patients with lithium-induced polyuria resulted in both a decreased urine output and increased urine osmolality. Thus, this treatment is more specific and safer than the previous use of thiazide diuretics, which might deplete both sodium and potassium (Battle et al., 1985). Lithium-induced nephrogenic diabetes insipidus is usually reversible, but several cases have been reported of its long persistence even after lithium has been stopped. Although the kidney tubule seems to be most vulnerable to lithium, the glomerulus has been involved in a few cases of minimal-change glomerulopathy with nephrotic syndrome (Moskovitz et al., 1981).

Patients receiving lithium should avoid dehydration with the consequent increased concentration of lithium in urine. Periodic monitoring with tests for renal concentrating ability are also a way to detect possible trouble. The renal toxicity of lithium has been extensively reviewed elsewhere (Hansen, 1981).

## Metabolic–Endocrine

The metabolic–endocrine effects of lithium were recently reviewed (Salata and Klein, 1987). Weight gain is frequent in lithium-treated patients and is probably a direct effect of the drug. Of 21 lithium-treated patients, 13 showed a gain of 5 percent total body weight when observed over a 12-month period. Only 2 of 12 placebo-treated patients had a similar degree of weight gain (Peselow et al., 1980).

Thyroid complications of long-term lithium treatment are frequent and are of serious concern. Relatively few patients develop frank thyroid enlargement and fewer still show symptoms of hypothyroidism. Serum thyroxine ($T_4$) and serum thyroid-stimulating hormone (TSH) were followed in 430 patients treated continually with lithium for 1 to 6 years. Overall, $T_4$ showed a small decrease at 6 months but returned to pretreatment levels by 12 months. Thereafter, it rose paradoxically until after 6 years of treatment it had risen to levels 53 percent higher than baseline. TSH was significantly increased at 6 and 12 months and then returned to prelithium levels. Eight patients required thyroxine treatment for hypothyroidism, about 2 per 100 patient-years of exposure. Single deviant values of TSH and $T_4$ were also encountered, followed by normal values. Thus, treatment should not be started on the basis of a single deviant value (Maarbjerg et al., 1987).

Others have suggested determinations of serum free-$T_4$ levels as being more sensitive than TSH measurement for routine monitoring. Both values are reported in currently available thyroid screening tests, so it remains to be seen which will be more accurate (Kutcher and Gow, 1987). Painless thyroiditis has been assumed to be the cause of transient hyperthyroidism usually followed by hypothyroidism. Thyroid microsomal antibody titers may be elevated in such patients along with other laboratory evidence of thyroid abnormality. A reversal of the usual sequence, in which hyperthyroidism followed hypothyroidism, was found in a single instance (McDermott et al., 1986).

Hyperparathyroidism associated with lithium treatment is not due to adenoma and can be treated conservatively. It seems to be due to a shift in the feedback regulation of parathyroid secretion by serum calcium levels; higher levels are required in the presence of lithium to suppress hormone secretion (Shen and Sherrard, 1982).

## Cardiac

T-wave flattening and inversion occurs in about 20 to 30 percent of patients treated with lithium. More reports of sinus node dysfunction or sinoatrial arrest have appeared, making "sick sinus" syndrome an absolute contraindication for the use of lithium. Ventricular irritability is a new observation that may be of serious import; lithium should be avoided in patients with frequent premature ventricular contractions. Various cardiac conduction defects can accompany lithium treatment, suggesting that when these exist lithium should be used cautiously, if at all. Myocarditis from lithium is highly questionable (Brady and Horgan, 1988). Most patients can be treated with little concern about cardiac consequences.

## Skin

Transient maculopapular, acneiform, and follicular eruptions have been noted in lithium treatment. Some of these eruptions subside with temporary discontinuation of treatment and will not recur with its resumption. In other cases they recur promptly with resumption of treatment. The appearance of 12 cases of psoriasis for the first time during lithium treatment, as well as exacerbation in three others, suggested that lithium might be capable of inducing psoriasis in susceptible persons. The skin lesions were reversible (Deandrea et al., 1982).

## Miscellaneous

Diarrhea, edema, and disturbed sexual function are various problems encountered in lithium treatment. Diarrhea can be troublesome. Increasing frequency of dosing so that smaller individual doses are used or a switch to slow-release lithium preparations are possible treatment approaches. Edema may be related to sodium retention and be treated with diuretics. If so, one must be aware of their effect on serum lithium levels.

A single case in which acute respiratory failure occurred in a woman with chronic obstructive pulmonary disease led to an investigation of the effect of lithium on respiratory responses to mouth obstruction. These were diminished, indicating that lithium could be a respiratory depressant (Weiner et al., 1983). It is somewhat surprising that additional cases have not been reported.

Withdrawal symptoms of heightened anxiety, irritability, and emotional liability followed withdrawal of lithium in four patients. Questionnaire data from 110 defaulters from a lithium clinic tended to confirm this possibility (King and Hullin, 1983). On the other hand, these might have been early symptoms of the recrudescence of mania.

Lithium regularly produces leukocytosis. Rather than representing recruitment from the marginal pool of leukocytes, it represents increased granulocytopoiesis. This common side effect has been turned into a treatment for patients with leucopenias of various causes.

## Pregnancy

Lithium is probably the psychotherapeutic drug most clearly known to be teratogenic. Lithium should be utterly avoided during the first trimester of pregnancy, owing to the frequent occurrence of Ebstein's cardiac malformation in the fetus. If a woman has been treated inadvertently during early pregnancy, abortion should be considered. Treatment with lithium late in pregnancy is possible, but lithium levels may fall with an increasing glomerular filtration rate, and then rise abruptly at parturition when the glomerular filtration rate falls. Because lithium passes easily into milk, breast feeding should be avoided (Linden and Rich, 1983).

# LITHIUM TOXICITY

More instances of intoxication with lithium occur inadvertently during treatment than as the result of deliberate overdose. In one study, of 23 patients with intoxication, 21 developed it in the former way (Hansen and Amdisen, 1978). Water loss due to impaired renal ability to conserve water seemed to be a major predisposing factor. Renal insufficiency was present in 17 patients, 7 of whom did not regain full function. Two patients died, and 5 developed persisting neurologic sequelae. The latter may include cognitive impairment, movement disorders, seizures, cerebellar syndrome, and peripheral neuropathies (Sansone and Ziegler, 1985).

Plasma concentrations often will not correctly predict the severity of potential toxicity. Levels may be high early on, during mild or moderate symptoms of intoxication, and then low later on, during severe symptoms of intoxication. When coma or subcoma develops, the mortality may be as high as 50 percent. Death is due often to pulmonary complications, the result of exceedingly viscous secretions from the respiratory tract, which are difficult to remove.

Although nausea and vomiting as well as diarrhea are common early signs of toxicity, they are quickly superseded by the numerous neurologic signs of toxicity. Lethargy and weakness may be followed by decreasing levels of consciousness. Tremors, myoclonic movements, increased muscle tonus, increased deep tendon reflexes, plantar extensor responses, and seizures may accompany decreasing consciousness. Death may also follow cardiac arrhythmias; at least in one instance postmortem examination revealed myocarditis and pericarditis.

After a deliberate overdose, the primary consideration is to rid the patient of the drug. Because of the physically large amounts of drug involved (one may be dealing with 30 to 60 g), absorption is slow. In part, this may be due to decreased gastrointestinal motility associated with impaired consciousness. Lavage should be done with a wide-bore tube, as the material tends to clump and may be difficult to remove through smaller tubes. Saline cathartics should follow lavage. Charcoal is not an effective absorbent in this instance; the use of cation exchange resins is theoretically possible.

Increasing excretion of lithium by forced alkaline diuretics, water diuretics, such as theophylline, or osmotic diuretics, such as mannitol, has occasionally been effective, but not much reliance can be placed on such measures. As lithium is a simple ion, it can be readily dialyzed. Hemodialysis should be carried out long enough to reduce the serum lithium concentration to less than 1 mEq/L.

Supportive measures include assisted respiration and maintained blood pressure, as in most poisonings, and monitoring of the electrocardiogram for the possible development of life-threatening arrhythmias. Special attention must be paid to the bronchial toilet, so that if viscous secretions develop, the patient does not asphyxiate. Serum lithium levels should be measured every 4 to 6 hours to assure that the measures are being successful in eliminating the drug. However, clinical observation of the patient takes precedence over lithium levels; some patients have shown decreasing consciousness even as their lithium concentrations are falling. The presence of seizures requires an anticonvulsant; either a loading dose of phenytoin or intravenous diazepam may be used.

# CARBAMAZEPINE

## History

Carbamazepine was first synthesized in the 1950s. In the 1960s and 1970s it was introduced into clinical practice as an anticonvulsant, first in Europe and then in the United States (Evans and Gualtieri, 1985). Carbamazepine was first used for manic-depressive illness in 1971, because of a hypothesized similarity between the rhythmic mood alterations of manic-depressive illness and the epileptiform discharges of epilepsy (Takezaki and Hanaoka, 1971). Since then, double-blind trials have substantiated this claim. Although many still consider lithium the only first-line treatment for manic-depressive illness, carbamazepine is considered to be an equivalent alternative.

## Pharmacology

### Pharmacokinetics

The absorption of carbamazepine from the gastrointestinal tract is slow. The attainment of peak serum levels can be highly variable (2 to 12 hours); its half-life is relatively long (31 to 35 hours). Protein binding is approximately 70 to 80 percent. Achieving stable therapeutic serum concentrations of carbamazepine can be complicated by the fact that the drug can increase its own metabolism by hepatic enzymes. Thus, it may take several days to select a daily dose that maintains therapeutic serum levels (4 to 12 $\mu$g/ml). The relationship between dose and plasma levels is poor (Levy and Kerr, 1988).

Metabolism of carbamazepine occurs via oxidation, first to a $-10,11$-epoxide metabolite and then to the $-10,11$-dihydroxide (see Fig. 6-3). One-third of the $-10,11$-dihydroxide is then conjugated as the glucuronide and eliminated; two-thirds is eliminated in the free form. The drug is excreted in both the urine and feces (Rodin, 1983). It should be noted that the $-10,11$-epoxide has potent anticonvulsant activity. Interestingly, in depressed patients, plasma concentrations of the $-10,11$-epoxide metabolite but not the parent compound have correlated with clinical efficacy (Post et al., 1983).

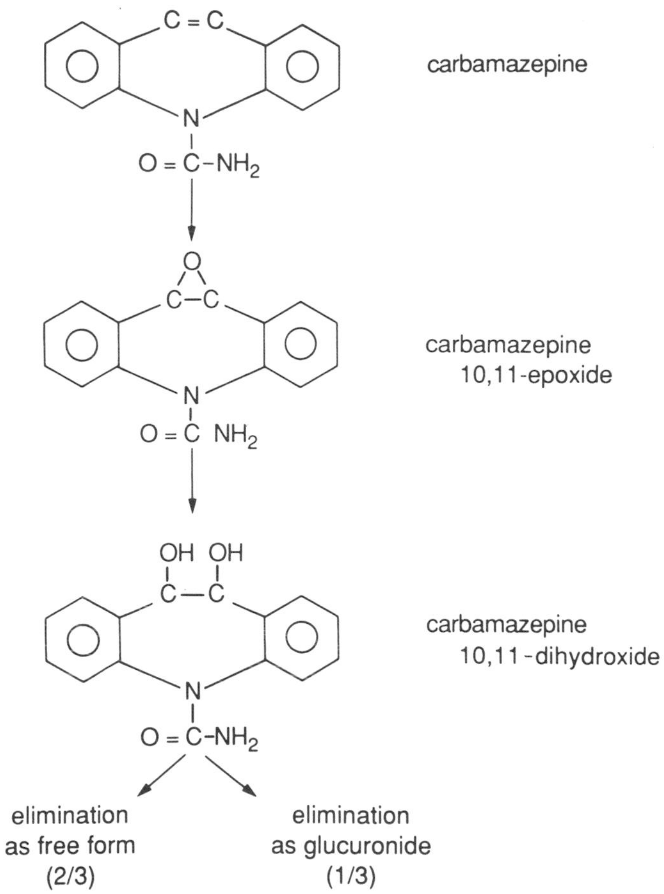
C = C
N
O = C-NH2
carbamazepine
O
C-C
N
O = C NH2
carbamazepine
10,11-epoxide
OH OH
C—C
N
O = C-NH2
carbamazepine
10,11-dihydroxide
elimination
as free form
(2/3)
elimination
as glucuronide
(1/3)

**Fig. 6-3.** Metabolism of carbamazepine.

## Mechanisms of Action

The discovery of carbamazepine as an effective drug for manic-depressive illness has added only further complexity to our attempts to understand the pathogenesis of manic-depressive illness. Like lithium, it has a multitude of pharmacologic actions, which vary on the basis of acute versus chronic administration. Possible mechanisms of action have been the subject of recent reviews (Evans and Gualtieri, 1985; Post, 1987; Elphick, 1988).

Carbamazepine interacts with sodium channels, dampening the influx of sodium ion into neurons (Worley and Baraban, 1987). As this action would have a stabilizing effect on synaptic transmission, this may be the basis of carbamazepine's efficacy as an anticonvulsant and in the treatment of trigeminal neuralgia. As one would expect for any tricyclic, carbamazepine blocks the reuptake of norepinephrine, although it has only 25 percent the activity of imipramine (Purdy et al., 1977). This action may contribute to its efficacy as an anticonvulsant, as the destruction of norepinephrine neurons will block the anticonvulsant effects of carbamazepine (Post, 1987). Moreover, this action may well explain its antidepressant effects in both bipolar and unipolar depression.

Carbamazepine (1) enhances the release and (2) blocks the reuptake of dopamine (Baros et al., 1986). It does not bind to or block postsynaptic dopamine receptors, however. This presynaptic effect on dopamine may be linked to the fact that in animals carbamazepine is capable of blocking neuroleptic-induced dopamine receptor increases.

Carbamazepine is a competitive adenosine antagonist (Marangos et al., 1985). However, whether this pharmacologic action is related to efficacy in manic-depressive illness awaits elucidation of adenosine's functions as a neuro-transmitter.

# CLINICAL USE OF CARBAMAZEPINE
## General

The growing popularity of carbamazepine as a treatment for manic-depressive illness and other related disorders seems to justify an in-depth discussion of its pharmacology and clinical use. In a large double-blind trial comparing car-bamazepine and chlorpromazine, its efficacy overall was equivalent to what one would expect of lithium. About 70 percent of manic patients responded (Okuma et al., 1979). Carbamazepine has prophylactic effects in manic-depressive illness as well (Kishimoto et al., 1983; Post et al, 1983). Carbamazepine and lithium should not be considered mutually exclusive treatments. In fact, in some cases of mania, concurrent administration of carbamazepine and lithium may be superior to treatment with either agent alone.

## Dose, Dosage, and Serum Levels

Clinical use of carbamazepine for manic-depressive illness follows guidelines similar as to when it is used for epilepsy. One should begin carbamazepine treatment with a dosage schedule of 200 mg twice a day. The daily dose may be increased in increments of 200 mg until a daily dose of 600 to 800 mg/day is achieved. Serum levels should be assessed 5 or 6 days after this dose has been reached, and additional dose increments can be performed as required. Most patients will require a dose of no more than 1200 mg/day. As noted earlier, carbamazepine may induce its own metabolism; thus, the daily dose may require further adjustment for several days.

In studies of carbamazepine for the treatment of manic-depressive illness, the daily dose has ranged broadly from 600 to 2000 mg/day, producing serum levels of 3 to 14 $\mu$g/ml. However, in the treatment of epilepsy as well as manic-depressive illness, it has been difficult to demonstrate correlations between serum levels and the degree of the clinical antimanic response (Post et al., 1987). At least as it regards the treatment of manic-depressive illness, this should not be surprising given the large number of clinical variables that may influence response. Some experts recommend that the daily dose of carbamazepine should be increased without regard to serum levels until intolerable side effects are encountered or until the dose reaches 2000 mg/day. In the classic Japanese studies, lower daily doses of carbamazepine were employed (approximately 500 mg/day), but these doses produced serum levels generally felt to be within the necessary range (3 to 12 $\mu$g/ml) (Okuma et al., 1979).

## Evaluating the Response to Carbamazepine

The overall response rate of patients with mania to carbamazepine is equivalent to that of lithium, that is, approximately 70 percent. Patients with mania should respond within 5 to 7 days of achieving therapeutic serum levels of carbamazepine. When carbamazepine is used to treat bipolar depression, however, one should expect to wait 2 or 3 weeks for a response. Carbamazepine is an effective treatment for prophylaxis in manic-depressive illness as well (Kishimoto et al., 1983; Post et al., 1983), blocking both depressive and manic episodes. The rate of efficacy for this use again appears equivalent to lithium (50 to 70 percent). Yet, additional clinical data should be obtained before definite conclusions are drawn.

The fact that lithium and carbamazepine have similar overall rates of efficacy in manic-depressive patients should not be construed to mean that they are interchangeable in individual patients. The clinical profile of the patient who benefits from carbamazepine may differ from that of a lithium responder. In one study, predictors of a good antimanic response to carbamazepine were (1) greater severity of manic symptoms, (2) anxiety and dysphoria, (3) a history of rapid cycling, and (4) a negative family history for manic-depressive illness (Post et al., 1987). Certainly, it makes good clinical sense that patients who are lithium failures should be tried on carbamazepine. Furthermore, many patients cannot tolerate one or more of lithium's many side effects. In these cases, a proper trial of lithium may not be possible, and carbamazepine may be highly useful.

## Other Indications for Carbamazepine

Like lithium, carbamazepine has been touted to have positive effects in the violent patient, regardless of the underlying diagnosis (Luchins, 1983). No data from controlled clinical trials are available to evaluate this possibility, and the difficulty of conducting proper studies for such an indication cannot be underestimated. Violence among psychiatric patients is hardly a homogeneous phenomenon, even among those who share the same diagnosis; treatment is usually most successful when the underlying brain disorder is the proximate cause of the violent behavior.

Carbamazepine should probably be expected to be an effective antidepressant, even in unipolar patients. This would follow logically from its effects on norepinephrine uptake. Its use in patients with personality disorders and mood instability is also being explored; however, insufficient clinical data preclude conclusions.

## Drug Interactions

Clinically significant interactions between carbamazepine and other drugs are few. The one of greatest concern is a pharmacodynamic interaction, in which the combination of carbamazepine with lithium increases neurotoxicity. Although a number of drugs (such as cimetidine, erythromycin, isoniazid, and propoxyphene) may increase plasma concentrations of carbamazepine, seldom is toxicity attributed to such an interaction. The same is true for a decreased plasma concentration with concurrent use of phenobarbital (Csernansky and Whiteford, 1987).

# ADVERSE EFFECTS
## Central Nervous System

Approximately one-third of patients treated with carbamazepine will experience side effects. The most commonly encountered side effects are related to the central nervous system, namely sedation, nausea, weakness, ataxia, diplopia, and mild nystagmus (Schmidt, 1982). These side effects are dose-dependent and may be avoided by a dose reduction. Subtle interference with a variety of cognitive processes, such as memory or attention, may also occur, even when clear-cut sedation is absent (Evans and Gualtieri, 1985).

Although carbamazepine is intended for its antipsychotic effects in manic patients, the opposite may occasionally occur. Case histories of patients treated for epilepsy who develop confusion or hallucinations have been reported (Silverstein et al., 1982). Thus far, no patients treated for manic-depressive illness with carbamazepine have had such side effects. Cases of dystonia (Jacome, 1979) and orofacial dyskinesia (Joyce and Gunderson, 1980) have also been reported in epilepsy patients taking carbamazepine. This should not be unexpected given the effects of the drug on dopamine reuptake and release.

## Blood Dyscrasias

Carbamazepine is known to produce leukopenia. In many cases this side effect is of a mild degree and spontaneously reversible and should not constitute an absolute contraindication for further therapy. In other cases, leukopenia may be irreversible and life-threatening. The drug should be immediately discontinued in these cases. Because leukopenia usually occurs early in treatment, a reasonable precaution is to obtain weekly leukocyte counts for the first 4 weeks of treatment and to discontinue treatment if a steadily progressive decrease in the leukocyte count occurs or if the leukocyte count falls below 4,000/mm$^3$ on any occasion.

## Pregnancy Complications

Because lithium is contraindicated during pregnancy, it may be tempting to substitute carbamazepine. Unfortunately, anticonvulsants should also be avoided during pregnancy if possible. In pregnant women treated for epilepsy with a variety of drugs, teratogenic malformations are more common, beginning with those that are relatively more common in the general population, such as cardiac abnormalities and cleft lip. A specific fetal antiepileptic drug syndrome has also been described, constituted by mental retardation, craniofacial abnormalities, and limb hypoplasias (Jones et al., 1989).

## Other Side Effects

Various types of skin eruptions have been reported with carbamazepine, ranging from urticaria to toxic epidermal necrolysis. Most seem to be allergic in origin and may respond to corticosteroids and cessation of treatment. Hepatitis, due to a direct toxic action on the liver as well as to hypersensitivity, is a rare complication. It may be heralded by anorexia, nausea, vomiting, and fever (Moore et al., 1985).

## OVERDOSE

Carbamazepine overdose is potentially life-threatening. The initial symptoms are drowsiness and ataxia, associated with plasma concentrations of 11 to 15 $\mu$g/ml. As plasma concentrations rise to 15 to 25 $\mu$g/ml, combativeness, hallucinations, and choreiform movements may follow. Levels above 25 $\mu$g/ml are associated with severe disturbance of consciousness, often coma. Coma usually lasts less than 24 hours. If seizures develop, intravenous diazepam or phenytoin may be used. As is often the case with overdoses of drugs that diminish gastrointestinal motility, late relapse has been observed, presumably owing to mobilization of unabsorbed drug. Although neurotoxic effects predominate, cardiotoxicity may be manifested by prolonged conduction and repolarization times. Cardiopulmonary arrest is a potential cause of death.

The kinetics of the drug change during massive overdose. Half-life is prolonged and the epoxide metabolite increases, presumably contributing to toxicity. The usual methods are used for trying to rid the body of drug, such as repeated oral gastric lavage followed by charcoal administration. Use of cathartics may spread the drug through the gastrointestinal tract and defeat the purposes of lavage. Although the drug has a large volume of distribution, charcoal hemoperfusion may be considered. Supportive measures should include close cardiac monitoring and management of electrolyte abnormalities. Seizures may be treated as mentioned previously. In short, many of the same principles of management are used as with overdoses of tricyclic antidepressants (May, 1984; Weaver et al., 1988).

# EXPERIMENTAL TREATMENTS

A variety of different approaches to treating manic-depressive disorder, other than lithium or carbamazepine, are currently under investigation. It is still too early to determine whether or not any will prove to be clinically useful.

## Valproate Sodium

The first use of valproate sodium in treating mania was reported in an article published in French in 1968. Because of the obscurity of the publication, not much attention was paid to this report. In 1980, an article published in English from a German clinic reported favorably on valproate in mania (Emrich et al., 1980). A review published in 1987 listed many individual reports but still covered relatively few cases, often poorly described with only a handful observed in any controlled fashion (McElroy et al., 1987). In addition, valproate has been tried in schizophrenia and in schizoaffective disorders. With increasing interest, the proper place of this drug in treatment should be exposed during the next several years.

## Clonazepam

Clonazepam, a benzodiazepine anticonvulsant, has little in common pharmacologically with either carbamazepine or valproate. It, too, has been reported to be effective for controlling mania (Chouinard et al., 1983). Whether such control is due to a direct antimanic action or whether the large doses used (12 to 16 mg/day) controlled the behavior by simple sedation is still unresolved.

## Verapamil

The calcium channel blocking drug verapamil has been reported to be efficacious in mania. In a sequential study, the drug was as effective as lithium and both were more effective than placebo. However, the design was inadequate and the number of patients treated were few (Giannini et al., 1984). As calcium influx is a requirement for the release of many neurotransmitters, it is presumed that decreasing release of a neurotransmitter, say dopamine, might be the basis for its effect.

## Clonidine

The alpha-2 adrenoreceptor agonist clonidine has had a checkered history as a psychotherapeutic drug. Five of 24 patients newly hospitalized for mania experienced complete responses to doses of 450 and 900 $\mu$g/day; another 5 patients had partial responses. Responses became evident 5 to 13 days after treatment (Hardy et al., 1986). A comparison between clonidine and verapamil, however, indicated that the latter drug was better (Giannini et al., 1985). Clonidine was first tried in the 1960s for treating schizophrenics; it seems never to lack for some psychiatric indication or other.

# REFERENCES

Albrecht J, Kampf D, Muller-Oerlinghausen B (1980) Renal function and biopsy in patients on lithium therapy. Pharmacopsychiatrie 13:228–234

Amdisen A (1987) The history of lithium. Biol Psychiatry 22:522–524

Angst J, Grof P (1976) The course of monopolar depressions and bipolar psychoses. pp 93–103. In Villeneuve A (ed): Lithium in Psychiatry: A Synopsis. Les Presses de L'Universite Laval, Quebec

Baron M, Risch N, Hamburger R, et al (1987) Genetic linkage between X-chromosome markers and bipolar affective illness. Nature 326:289–292

Baros HMT, Braz S, Leite JR (1986) Effect of carbamazepine on dopamine release and reuptake in rat striatal slices. Epilepsia 27(5):534–537

Battle DC, von Riotte AB, Gaviril M, Grupp M (1985) Amelioration of polyuria by amiloride in patients receiving long-term lithium therapy. N Engl J Med 312:408–414

Biederman J, Lerner Y, Belmaker RH (1979) Combination of lithium carbonate and haloperidol in schizo-affective disorder. Arch Gen Psychiatry 36:327–333

Brady HR, Horgan JH (1988) Lithium and the heart; unanswered questions. Chest 92:166–169

Brockington IF, Kendell BE, Wainwright S, et al (1979) The distinction between the affective psychoses and schizophrenia. Br J Psychiatry 135:243–248

Cade JFJ (1970) The story of lithium. pp 218–229. In Ayd FJ Jr, Blackwell B (eds): Biological Psychiatry. JB Lippincott, Philadelphia

Cameron OG, Smith CB (1980) Comparison of acute and chronic lithium treatment on 3H-norepinephrine uptake by rat brain slices. Psychopharmacology (Berlin) 67:81–85

Chouinard G, Young SN, Annable L (1983) Antimanic effect of clonazepam. Biol Psychiatry 18:451–466.

Colburn RW, Goodwin FK, Bunney WE Jr, Davis JM (1967) Effect of lithium on the uptake of noradrenaline by synaptosomes. Nature 215:1395–1397.

Consensus Development Conference (1984) Mood Disorder: Pharmacologic Prevention of Recurrences. Vol 5, No 4. National Institutes of Health, Bethesda, Md

Cooper TB, Bergner PEE, Simpson GM (1973) The 24-hour serum lithium level as a prognosticator of dosage requirements. Am J Psychiatry 130:601–603

Coppen A, Abou-Saleh M, Milln P, et al (1983) Decreasing lithium dosage reduces morbidity and side effects during prophylaxis. J Affective Disord 5:353–362

Craft M, Ismail IA, Krishnamurti D, et al (1987) Lithium in the treatment of aggression in mentaly handicapped patients. A double-blind trial. Br J Psychiatry 150:685–689

Csernansky JG, Whiteford HA (1987) Clinically significant psychoactive drug interactions. pp 802–815. In Hales RE, Frances AJ (eds): American Psychiatric Association Annual Review, Vol 6. American Psychiatric Press, Inc, Washington DC

Deandrea D, Walker N, Mehlmauer M, White K (1982) Dermatological reactions to lithium: a critical review of the literature. J Clin Psychopharmacol 2:199–204

Derby IM (1933) Manic-depressive "exhaustion" deaths. Psychiatric 7:436–449

Diagnostic and Statistical Manual of Mental Disorders, 3rd ed, DSM-III. American Psychiatric Association, Washington DC, 1980, pp 208–210

Egeland JA, Gerhard DS, Pauls DL, et al (1987) Bipolar affective disorders linked to DNA markers on chromosome 11. Nature 325:783–787.

Elphick M (1988) The clinical uses and pharmacology of carbamazepine in psychiatry. Int Clin Psychopharmacol 3:185–203

Emrich HM, Zerssen D, Kissling W, et al (1980) Effects of sodium valproate on mania. The GABA-hypothesis of affective disorders. Arch Psychiatr Nervenkr 229:1–16

Evans RW, Gualtieri CT (1985) Carbamazepine: a neuropsychological and psychiatric profile. Clin Neuropharmacol 8:221–241

Fawcett J, Kravitz HM (1985) The long-term management of bipolar disorders with lithium, carbamazepine and antidepressants. J Clin Psychiatry 46:58–60

Fawcett J, Clark DC, Aagensen CA (1987) A double-blind placebo-controlled trial of lithium carbonate therapy for alcoholism. Arch Gen Psychiatry 44:248–256

Gershon ES, Delisi E, Hamovit J et al (1988) A controlled family study of chronic psychoses. Arch Gen Psychiatry 45:328–336

Giannini AJ, Houser WL Jr, Loiselle RH, et al (1984) Antimanic effects of verapamil. Am J Psychiatry 141:1602–1603

Giannini AJ, Loiselle RH, Price WA, Giannini MC (1985) Comparison of antimanic efficacy of clonidine and verapamil. J Clin Pharmacol 25:307–308

Goodnick PJ, Fieve RR, Meltzer HL, Dunner DL (1981) Lithium elimination half-life and duration of therapy. Clin Pharmacol Ther 29:47–50

Groth U, Prellwitz W, Jahnchen E (1974) Estimation of pharmacokinetic parameters of lithium from saliva and urine. Clin Pharmacology Ther 16:490–498

Hansen HE (1981) Renal toxicity of lithium. Drugs 22:461–476

Hansen HE, Amdisen A (1978) Lithium intoxication (report of 23 cases and review of 100 cases from the literature.) Q J Med 47:123–144

Hardy MC, Lecrubier Y, Widlocher D (1986) Efficacy of clonidine in 24 patients with acute mania. Am J Psychiatry 143:1450–1453.

Helmar O, Rafaelsen OJ (1987) Lithium: long-term effects on the kidney. IV. Renal lithium clearance. Acta Psychiatr Scand 76:193–198

Hestbech J, Hansen HE, Amdisen A, Olsen S (1977) Chronic renal lesions following long-term treatment with lithium. Kidney Int 12:250–213

Himmelhoch JM, Forrest J, Neil JF, Detre TP (1977) Thiazide-lithium synergy in recurrent affective disorders. Psychiatry 134:149–152

Hirschowitz J, Casper R, Garver DL, Chang S (1980) Lithium response in good prognosis schizophrenia. Am J Psychiatry 137(8):916–920

Hodgkinson S, Sherrington S, Gurling H, et al (1987) Molecular genetic evidence for heterogeneity in manic depression. Nature 325:805–806

Jacome D (1979) Carbamazepine-induced dystonia. JAMA 241(21): 2263 (Letter to the editor)

Janowsky DS, El-Yousef K, Davis JM, Sekerke HJ (1972) A cholinergic–adrenergic hypothesis of mania and depression. Lancet 2:632–635

Jefferson JW, Greist JH (1981) Some hazards of lithium use. Am J Psychiatry 138:93

Jones KL, Lacro RV, Johnson KA, Adams J (1989) Pattern of malformation in the children of women treated with carbamazepine during pregnancy. N Engl J Med 320:1661–1666

Joyce RP, Gunderson CH (1980) Carbamazepine-induced orofacial dyskinesia. Neurology 30:1333–1334

King JR, Hullin RP (1983) Withdrawal symptoms from lithium. Four case reports and a questionnaire study. Br J Psychiatry 143:30–35

Kishimoto A, Ogura C, Hazama H, Inoue K (1983) Long-term prophylactic effects of carbamazepine in affective disorder. Br J Psychiatry 143:327–331.

Kline NS, Wren JC, Cooper TB, et al (1974) Evaluation of lithium therapy in chronic and periodic alcoholism. Am J Med Sci 268:15–22

Kutcher SP, Gow SM (1987) Free $T_4$ measurement is preferred to the $T_4$ test for thyroid evaluation in lithium treated patients. Can J Psychiatry 32:112–114

Levy RH, Kerr BM (1988) Clinical pharmacokinetics of carbamazepine. J Clin Psychiatry 49 (4, suppl):58–61

Linden S, Rich CL (1983) The use of lithium during pregnancy and lactation. J Clin Psychiatry 44:358–361

Luchins DJ (1983) Carbamazepine for the violent psychiatric patient. Lancet 1:766

Maarbjerg K, Vestergaard P, Schou M (1987) Changes in serum thyroxine ($T_4$) and serum thyroid-stimulating hormone (TSH) during prolonged lithium treatment. Acta Psychiatr Scand 75:217–221

Mander AJ, Loudon JB (1988) Rapid recurrence of mania following abrupt discontinuation of lithium. Lancet 2:15–17

Marangos PJ, Weiss SRB, Montgomery P, et al (1985) Chronic carbamazepine treatment increases brain adenosine receptors. Epilepsia 26(5):493–498

May DC (1984) Acute carbamazepine intoxication: clinical spectrum and management. South Med J 77:24–26

McDermott MT, Burman KD, Hofeldt FD, Kidd GS (1986) Lithium-associated thyrotoxicosis. Am J Med 80:1245–1248

McElroy SL, Keck PE Jr, Pope HG Jr (1987) Sodium valproate: its use in primary psychiatric disorders. J Clin Psychopharmacol 7:16–24

Meltzer HL (1986) Lithium mechanisms in bipolar illness and altered intracellular calcium functions. Biol Psychiatry 21:492–510

Mendlewiez J, Simon P, Sevy S, et al (1987) Polymorphic DNA marker on X-chromosome and manic-depression. Lancet 1:1230–1234

Menkes HA, Baraban JM, Freed AN, Snyder SH (1986) Lithium dampens neurotransmitter response in smooth muscle: relevance to action in affective illness. Proc Nat Acad Sci USA 83.

Moore NC, Lever B, Meyendorff E, Gershon S (1985) Three cases of carbamazepine toxicity. Am J Psychiatry 142:974–975

Moskovitz, R, Springer P, Urquhart M (1981) Lithium-induced nephrotic syndrome. Am J Psychiatry 138:382–383

Muller-Oerlinghausen B (1985) Lithium longterm treatment: does it act via serotonin? Pharmacopsychiatry 18:214–217

Nelson JC (1986) Lithium augmentation in psychotic depression refractory to combined drug treatment. Am J Psychiatry 143:363–366

Nielsen-Kudsk F, Amdisen A (1979) Analysis of the pharmacokinetics of lithium in man. Eur J Pharmacol 16:271–277

Okuma T, Inanaga K, Otsuki S (1979) Comparison of the antimanic efficacy of carbamazepine and chlorpromazine: a double-blind controlled study. Psychopharmacology 66:211–217

Peselow ED, Dunner DL, Fieve RR, Lautin A (1980) Lithium carbonate and weight gain. J Affective Disord 2:303–310

Petursson H (1979) Prediction of lithium response. Compr Psychiatry 20:226–241

Post RM (1987) Mechanisms of action of carbamazepine and related anticonvulsants in affective illness. pp 567–576. In Meltzer HY (ed): Psychopharmacology: The Third Generation of Progress. Raven Press, New York

Post RM, Jimerson DC, Bunney WE Jr, Goodwin FK (1980) Dopamine and mania: behavioral and biochemical effects of the dopamine receptor blocker pimozide. Psychopharmacology 67:297–305.

Post RM, Uhde TW, Ballenger JC, et al (1983) Carbamazepine and its −10,11-epoxide metabolite in plasma and CSF. Arch Gen Psychiatry 40:673–676

Post RM, Uhde TW, Ballenger JC, Squillace KM (1983) Prophylactic efficacy of carbamazepine in manic-depressive illness. Am J Psychiatry 140:1602–1604

Post RM, Uhde TW, Ry-Byrne R, Joffe RT (1987) Correlates of antimanic response to carbamazepine. Psychiatry Res 21:71–83

Prien RF, Caffey EM Jr, Klett CJ (1972) A comparison of lithium carbonate and chlorpromazine in the treatment of excited schizo-affectives. Arch Gen Pschiatry 27:182–189

Purdy RE, Julien RM, Fairhurst AS, Terry MD (1977) Effect of carbamazepine on the in vitro uptake and release of norepinephrine in adrenergic nerves of rabbit aorta and in whole brain synaptosomes. Epilepsia 18(2):251–257

Reimann IW, Frohlich JC (1981) Effects of diclofenac on lithium kinetics. Clin Pharmacol Ther 30:348–352.

Rieder RO, Mann LS, Weinberger DR, et al (1983) Computed tomographic scans in patients with schizophrenia, schizoaffective, and bipolar affective disorder. Arch Gen Psychiatry 40:735–739

Rodin EA (1983) Carbamazepine (Tegretol). pp. 203–213. In Brown TR, Feldman RG (eds): Epilepsy Diagnosis and Managment. Little Brown, Boston

Rosenberg JG, Binder RL, Berlant J (1987) Prediction of therapeutic lithium dose: comparison and improvement of current methods. J Clin Pscyhiatry 48:284–286

Salata R, Klein I (1987) Effects of lithium on the endocrine system: review. J Lab Clin Med 110:130–136.

Samiy AH, Rosnick PB (1987) Early identification of renal problems in patients receiving chronic lithium treatment. Am J Pscyhiatry 144:670–672

Sansone ME, Ziegler DK (1985) Lithium toxicity: a review of neurologic complications. Clin neuropharmacol 8:242–248

Schmidt D (1982) Adverse Effects of Antiepileptic Drugs. Raven Press, New York

Schou M (1957) Biology and pharmacology of lithium ion. Pharmacol Rev 9:17–58

Schou M (1988) Lithium treatment of manic-depressive illness. Past, present and perspectives. JAMA 259:1834–1836

Schuckit MA (1986) Genetic and clinical implications of alcoholism and affective disorder. Am J Psychiatry 143:140–147

Shen FH, Sherrard DJ (1982) Lithium-induced hyperparathyroidism: an alteration of the "set-point." Ann Intern Med 96:63–65

Sherman WR, Leavitt AL, Honchar MP, et al (1981) Evidence that lithium alters phosphoinostitide metabolism: chronic administration elevates primarily D-myo-inositolophosphate in cerebral cortex of the rat. Neurochem 36(6):1947–1951

Silverstein FS, Parrish MA, Johnston MV (1982) Clinical and laboratory observations. Adverse behavioral reactions in children treated with carbamazepine (Tegretol). J Pediatr 101(5):785–787

Simard M, Gumbiner B, Lee A, et al (1989) Lithium carbonate intoxication. A case report and review of the literature. Arch Intern Med 149:36–46

Snider RM, Fisher SK, Agranoff BW (1987) Inositide-linked second messengers in the central nervous system. pp. 317–324. In Meltzer HY (ed): Psychopharmacology: The Third Generation of Progress. Raven Press, New York

Spring GK (1979) Neurotoxicity with combined use of lithium and thioridazine. J Clin Psychiatry 40:135–138.

Stokes PE, Kocsis JH, Arcuni OJ (1976) Relationship of lithium chloride dose to treatment response in acute mania. Arch Gen Psychiatry 33:1080–1084

Swann AC, Berman N, Frazer A, et al (1987) Lithium distribution in mania; plasma and red blood cell lithium, clinical state and monoamine metabolites during lithium treatment. Psychiatry Res 20:1–12

Takezaki H, Hanaoka M (1971) The use of carbamazepine (Tegretol) in the control of manic depressive psychosis and other manic depressive states. J Clin Psychiatry 13:173–183.

Thornhill DP (1981) The biological disposition and kinetics of lithium. Biopharm Drug Disposition 2:305–322

Treiser SL, Cascio CS, O'Donohue TL, et al (1981) Lithium increases serotonin release and decreases serotonin receptors in the hippocampus. Science 213:1529–1531

Tyrer P, Alexander MS, Regan A, Lee I (1980) An extrapyramidal syndrome after lithium therapy. Br J Psychiatry 136:191–194.

Vestergaard P, Amdisen A, Shou M (1980) Clinically significant side effects of lithium treatment. A survey of 237 patients in long-term treatment. Acta Psychiatr Scand 62:193–200

Wahlin A, Bucht G, Von Knorring L, Smigan L (1980) Kidney function in patients with affective disorders with and without lithium therapy. Int Pharmacopsychiatr 5: 253–259

Weaver DF, Camfield P, Fraser A (1988) Massive carbamazepine overdose: clinical and pharmacologic observations in five episodes. Neurology 38:755–759

Wehr TA, Goodwin FK (1987) Can antidepressants cause mania and worsen the course of affective illness? Am J Psychiatry 144:1403–1411

Wehr TA, Sack D, Rosenthal N, et al (1983) Circadian rhythm disturbances in manic-depressive illness. Fed Proc 42:2809–2814

Weiner M, Chausow A, Wolpert E, et al (1983) Effect of lithium on the responses to added respiratory resistance. N Engl J Med 308:319–321

Wood AJ, Goodwin GM (1987) A review of the biochemical and neuropharmacological actions of lithium. Psychol Med 17:579–600

Worley PF, Baraban JM (1987) Site of anticonvulsant action on sodium channels: autoradiographic and electrophysiological studies in rat brain. Proc Nat Acad Sci USA 84:3051–3055

# 7

# PSYCHOTHERAPEUTIC DRUGS FOR CHILDREN AND ADOLESCENTS

Psychotherapeutic drugs are increasingly used to treat children and adolescents. In addition, a major shift has occurred in our attempts to diagnose and understand the nature of psychiatric disorders among the young. In keeping with the recent emphasis in adults on objective, empiric diagnostic criteria, there has been an aggressive attempt to define objectively the psychopathology of childhood. The *Diagnostic and Statistical Manual* of the American Psychiatric Association (DSM-IIIR, 1987) lists specific behavioral criteria for disorders relatively unique to children and adolescents (for example, separation anxiety disorder, attention-deficit hyperactivity disorder, autistic disorder) and also "permits" diagnostic criteria formulated for adult cases of psychosis and major mood disorders to be applied to children. The validation of these criteria, in particular those that are analogous to or drawn from adult disorders, remains the subject of ongoing research.

Pediatric psychopharmacology is a field in transition, from one in which drugs were avoided or used in a largely nonspecific manner to control maladaptive behavior to one in which drugs are used to manage specific biopsychological disorders based on plausible neurochemical rationales. More than 20 years ago, psychotherapeutic drug treatment in children was thought to play a very narrow role. Use of placebos to establish a baseline response or to check the response to drugs was recommended. Treatment might be considered only for a few days of each week and for as brief a period of time as possible. On the other hand, it was recognized that drugs could be helpful for appropriate indications and severe problems. Doses were recommended to be individualized, with precautions taken against adverse effects. Older drugs were preferred to newer ones unless the latter were clearly superior (Eisenberg, 1964; Werry, 1967). Later, these general principles were modified to indicate the need for an objective diagnosis and the possibility that treatment might have to be long-term (Werry, 1979).

159

Even today, wide variations in practice are encountered, from some pediatric psychiatrists who use drugs sparingly, if at all, to others who use them in a pattern similar to their use in adults.

The following discussion will first review drugs that may be useful for treating schizophrenia, mania, and depression in children. In each case, the clinician and researcher can ask to what extent these disorders in children are similar to the adult form, and whether an understanding of pharmacologic principles drawn from the study of adults should be applied to children. We will certainly highlight any known differences with adult psychopharmacology when applicable. Second, we will discuss the treatment of disorders that are relatively specific to childhood; these raise unique questions regarding the pathogenesis of psychopathology and the mechanisms of drug action.

Pediatric psychopharmacology remains a field in rapid growth. A great emphasis has developed on diagnosing, understanding, and treating childhood disorders with a biologic basis. In most cases, it is hoped that the systematic study of the effects of psychotherapeutic drugs will be a key element in shedding light on the pathogenesis of such disorders. A summary of current practices in using psychotherapeutic drugs in children and adolescents is found in Table 7-1.

# SCHIZOPHRENIA
## Diagnostic Considerations

The proper use of neuroleptics in children depends on accurate diagnosis. Until recently, the diagnostic boundary between childhood-onset schizophrenia and infantile autism was confused. In the 1940s, infantile autism was considered to be the earliest manifestation of schizophrenia. The distinct pattern of behaviors observed, such as extreme withdrawal and stereotypies, as well as the absence of common symptoms of psychosis, such as hallucinations and delusions, was attributed to the fact that the disease attacked the patient at a very early developmental stage. Thus, in the *Diagnostic and Statistical Manual,* Second Edition (DSM-II), special criteria were given for the diagnosis of childhood schizophrenia as contrasted to adult-onset schizophrenia, and no mention is made of infantile autism as a separate diagnostic entity.

Clinical research has recently revealed that childhood-onset schizophrenia and infantile autism can be distinguished on several grounds. They are phenomenologically distinct; classic symptoms of psychosis do occur in children that permit the use of adult criteria for the diagnosis of schizophrenia (Green et al., 1984). These two groups can also be differentiated based on demographic variables and intelligence. In fact, children with schizophrenia and infantile autism are similar only in that they both show severely disturbed interpersonal behaviors. In the DSM-IIIR, adult criteria are used to diagnose schizophrenia in children, and separate criteria are listed for the diagnosis of infantile autism.

Despite these advances, diagnosis of psychosis in childhood is imprecise. Some psychotic processes that begin at age 11 or 12 years may show only stormy behavior. Other children with autistic-like behavior may develop typical

**Table 7-1.** Psychotherapeutic Drugs in Children and Adolescents

Antidepressants, Tricyclic
   Primary indication: depression, any type
   Secondary indications: separation anxiety, enuresis, anorexia/bulimia
   Doses: 2–5 mg/kg/day for depression
      0.5–2.0 mg/kg/day enuresis

Antidepressants, MAO Inhibitors
   Primary indication: depression, phobias
   Secondary indications: anorexia/bulimia
   Doses: phenelzine, 1 mg/kg/day

Mood Stabilizers
   Primary indication: manic-depressive illness
   Secondary indications: conduct disorder, aggressive behavior
   Doses: lithium enough to produce serum concentration of 0.6–1.2 mEq/L
      carbamazepine            6–12 years            10 mg/kg/day divided

Antipsychotics
   Primary indication: schizophrenia, mania
   Secondary indications: mental retardation, autism, Tourette syndrome
   Doses: thioridazine 1.5–3.0 mg/kg/day
      chlorpromazine 1.5–3.0 mg/kg/day
      haloperidol 0.1–0.5 mg/kg/day
      pimozide 0.05–0.2 mg/kg/day (Tourette)

Anxiolytics/Hypnotics
   Primary indications: anxiety, any type; insomnia
   Secondary indications: separation anxiety, obsessive-compulsive disorder
   Doses: unexplored

Stimulants
   Primary indications: attention-deficit/hyperactivity, narcolepsy
   Doses: dextroamphetamine 2.5–40 mg/day
      methylphenidate 50–80 mg/day
      magnesium pemoline 6+ years 37.5–112.5 mg/day

symptoms of schizophrenia as they mature. During adolescence, some may develop an insidious onset of schizophrenic psychosis, similar to what may occur in adults. Others, however, may simply be diagnosed as "anxious" during late adolescence and only become frankly psychotic during early adult life. Schizophreniform psychoses may follow abuse of stimulants or follow other acute psychological stresses. They are often self-limiting. Thus, the diagnosis of psychosis or severe disturbed behavior in childhood is not always clear. One must sometimes proceed with treatment despite uncertainty.

## Responses to Treatment

The symptoms of childhood-onset schizophrenia usually remit after treatment with neuroleptics. Improvement is most apparent in patients with clear-cut, severe psychotic symptoms (Fish et al., 1966). As schizophrenia has an insidious onset in many children, the clinician is often challenged by the decision regarding when to begin neuroleptic treatment. It is not an uncommon experience to observe a child worsening gradually. Initial symptoms may be seclusiveness, disturbed relationships, or lack of concentration (Aakrog and Mortensen, 1985). Subtle forms of thought disorder may precede the onset of psychotic symptoms, and peculiarities of thought content may only border on the delusional (Parnas et al., 1982; Arboleda and Holzman, 1985). In such cases, one cannot know for certain that psychosis in the future is inevitable, and to proceed with a diagnosis of schizophrenia and begin administration of neuroleptics has obvious risks. Furthermore, there are few data to say whether treatment of schizophrenia during its initial prodrome will decrease or increase the severity of the overall course of illness.

Based on the foregoing discussion, neuroleptic treatment should be reserved for cases in which clear-cut psychotic symptoms have already emerged. The daily dose should be modest when treatment is begun and should be titrated downward during remission, so that clinicians may be certain that they are using the lowest dose necessary to control psychosis. Low potency neuroleptics, such as chlorpromazine or thioridazine, are quite sedative but are preferred by some owing to the lower incidence of extrapyramidal effects. High potency drugs, such as haloperidol, may produce acute dystonic reactions, especially in boys. It is, however, difficult to generalize about which antipsychotic may be most useful and best tolerated by individual children. A conservative approach to initial doses as well as covering patients treated with high potency drugs with antiparkinson drugs should minimize potential problems.

Long-term neuroleptic treatment can lead to the development of tardive dyskinesia in children, just as in adults. However, in cases of childhood-onset schizophrenia, spontaneous mannerisms and stereotypies occur frequently, which may be difficult to distinguish from the movements of tardive dyskinesia. For this reason, it is wise to obtain an objective record of abnormal movements in all children before the start of neuroleptic treatment (Campbell et al., 1983). Without such documentation, one might erroneously attribute spontaneous abnormal movements to neuroleptic treatment.

# DEPRESSION
## Diagnostic Considerations

As with childhood-onset schizophrenia, considerable controversy regarding the existence of childhood-onset depression has prevailed until recently (Angold, 1988). The classic psychoanalytic perspective viewed children as unable to manifest depression because of an undeveloped superego. However, as adult psychiatric diagnosis became rooted in the empiric description of symptoms and signs, a similar approach was applied to children. Cytryn and McKnew (1972) were among the first to describe the symptoms of depression in children in systematic terms and suggested a three-type classification: (1) acute depression, (2) chronic depression, and (3) masked depression. Later, these same investigators recognized that the adult criteria for depression, as put forward in DSM-III, could be used to diagnose depression in almost all children (Cytryn et al., 1980). Certainly children with depression may be brought to the clinician by parents who complain of behavioral problems suggestive of other diagnoses, such as conduct disorder. However, a careful history taken from the child himself will usually reveal the correct diagnosis (Carlson and Cantwell, 1980). The presence of certain vegetative signs (hypersomnia, increased appetite, psychomotor retardation) may be telling.

Depression in adolescents may be associated with other problems, such as learning disability, bulimia, or school refusal. Symptoms may be vague, such as a decrease in school performance, complaint of easy fatigue or various pains of uncertain cause, increasing irritability, or low self-esteem. The extent to which family history may be positive varies; one cannot rule out depression because of the absence of a family history.

The incidence of major depression among 9-year-old children in the general population of New Zealand, using Research Diagnostic Criteria similar to DSM-III criteria, was estimated to be 1.8 percent. Minor depression was found in an additional 2.5 percent (Kashani et al., 1983). Thus, mood disorders cannot be considered rare in childhood. Nor should they be considered as trivial. Suicides and suicidal attempts are well documented in children and even more so in adolescents. In the latter group, suicide ranks just behind accidents or homicides as a leading cause of death.

## Response to Treatment

The efficacy of tricyclic antidepressants in depressed children remains difficult to prove. Open-label studies have been suggestive (Puig-Antich et al., 1978). However, no double-blind studies have been able to substantiate a significant drug effect (Kramer and Feiguine, 1981; Kashani et al., 1984). This failure is likely due to the very small sample sizes used in such studies and a high rate of placebo response. Linear correlations have been found between the degree of clinical response and higher plasma drug concentrations, after placebo-responders were removed (Preskorn et al., 1982; Puig-Antich et al., 1979). The range of plasma imipramine (plus desipramine) concentrations required for an antidepressant response appear to be similar to those suggested for adults, that is, above 150 to 200 ng/ml. The doses of imipramine required to sustain such levels are 2 to 5 mg/kg day. Doses above 3.5 mg/day can be associated with cardiotoxicity, so patients should be carefully watched. Doses of more than 5 mg/day should not be used. In one study, the single-dose elimination rate for nortriptylin was similar in children compared to adults (Geller et al., 1984).

Although an early study indicated an antidepressant effect of phenelzine as compared with placebo in childhood depression, few subsequent studies have investigated the use of MAO inhibitors for this purpose (Frommer, 1967). Phenelzine has also been useful in treating anorexia nervosa.

# MANIC-DEPRESSIVE DISORDER
## Diagnostic Considerations

Anthony and Scott (1960) first suggested the possibility that manic-depressive illness might occur in children as well as in adults. Since then, numerous case reports have appeared. In two of these, the illness was reported to have begun at the age of 24 months (Feinstein and Wolpert, 1973), and 11-1/2 months (LaGrone, 1981). Weinberg and Brumback (1976) described five additional cases of childhood mania and suggested specific diagnostic criteria for the disorder. However, these criteria are so similar to those now listed in the DSM-IIIR for adults with mania, that the latter criteria may be used in most cases. At present, the occurrence of mania in children is no longer controversial.

Manifestations of mania in children may be erratic—shifting moods with intact intelligence, explosive outbursts, sleep disturbance, hyperphagia, encopresis, and cyclic episodes of depression. With regard to the differential diagnosis in such cases, one must consider attention-deficit disorder and schizophrenia. In addition to a careful history and mental status examination, a strong family history of manic-depressive illness may be highly revealing. Patients who may be misdiagnosed as having attention-deficit disorder are usually made worse by stimulant treatment, which provides a useful diagnostic clue.

## Response to Treatment

Several open label studies of lithium carbonate have been performed in children and adolescents. These suggest that lithium carbonate may be safely administered and is effective. Annell (1969) successfully treated 12 cases of mania with onset in adolescence. Gram and Rafaelsen (1972) had similarly good results in treating 11 cases, aged 8 to 22 years. In the largest series available, Youngerman and Canino (1978) reported that 30 out of 46 patients, aged 3 to 19 years, responded well to lithium carbonate. In general, prominent symptoms of a cyclic bipolar disorder and a strong family history of manic-depressive illness that responds favorably to lithium carbonate are the best predictors of a good clinical response in individual children.

Lithium dose and dosage should be essentially similar in children and adults. Brumback and Weinberg (1977) used doses of 30 to 40 mg/kg/day in six children and achieved stable serum concentrations of 0.6 to 1.2 mEq/L. Some adolescents may require higher than usual serum lithium concentrations to obtain an initial response. Doses should be lowered to attain more customary concentrations once remission is under way.

Failure to respond to lithium might indicate an alternative diagnosis. Lithium carbonate has shown little efficacy for the treatment of attention-deficit disorder with hyperactivity (Whitehead and Clark, 1970). However, not every case of manic-depressive illness is responsive to lithium. Also, lithium has nonspecific sedative and possibly antiaggressive effects. Thus, a beneficial response to lithium carbonate does not necessarily prove the diagnosis of manic-depressive illness. One assumes that carbamazepine, just as in adults, may be a suitable alternative to lithium.

## ANXIETY DISORDERS
### Diagnostic Considerations

Several specific childhood disorders are now described in the DSM-IIIR in which anxiety is a predominant symptom. These are (1) separation anxiety disorder, (2) avoidant disorder of childhood or adolescence, and (3) overanxious disorder. However, the validity of these syndromes, as well as the use of antianxiety drugs to treat anxiety in children and adolescents, remains largely unexplored. When faced with the anxious child, the clinician is more likely to examine and treat the child's environment, rather than to administer sedatives. This policy is sensible and has stood the test of time. Rarely does anxiety persist independently of identifiable family or peer problems in most children. In others, particularly adolescents, who are in the process of manifesting a personality disorder, anxiety may be chronic and free-floating. Whether anxiety in such patients exists alone, or represents a prodrome of schizophrenia or depression, is often unclear.

Little work has been done to determine whether panic disorder and related agoraphobia occur with a significant frequency in children and adolescents. The general impression has been that these disorders are rare in children, but panic disorders may be more common in adolescents. The symptoms may be confused with conduct disorder. Many such patients respond to tricyclics. On the other hand, obsessive-compulsive disorder is being identified in children and adolescents at an increasing rate. Consistent with this trend, approximately one-third of adults with obsessive-compulsive disorder report that their symptoms began before the age of 15 (Rapoport et al., 1981). When this disorder occurs in children, its manifestations are nearly identical to adult obsessive-compulsive disorder. Therefore, as with many other childhood disorders, DSM-IIIR adult criteria may be used for diagnosis.

### Response to Treatment

In an isolated and somewhat controversial study, Gittelman-Klein and Klein (1973) studied the effects of imipramine in 35 children between the ages of 6 and 14 who were phobic of school attendance. The dose administered ranged from 100 to 200 mg/day. Significant improvement in several areas was detected after 6 weeks of double-blind, placebo-controlled treatment. The child's willingness to separate from the mother increased, and physical symptoms in the school setting decreased. The patients' mothers reported a decrease in apparent depression. This study has not been replicated, possibly because the gains seemed to be slight compared with the risk of such high doses of a tricyclic antidepressant.

Clomipramine, a tricyclic antidepressant that blocks the neuronal reuptake of serotonin, has been found to be effective in treating obsessive-compulsive disorder in adults (Insel et al., 1983). Concomitant depression does not appear to be necessary for an improvement in obsessions and compulsions, and plasma levels of clomipramine appear to predict the degree of response. Such studies have led, in part, to hypotheses that an abnormality of serotonin neuro-transmission is involved in the pathogenesis of obsessive-compulsive disorder. Clomipramine is effective for the treatment of obsessive-compulsive disorder in children as well as in adults. Doses of 100 to 200 mg/day are well-tolerated in children, yielding plasma concentrations of 36 to 152 ng/ml (Flament et al., 1985).

Virtually no literature exists concerning use of benzodiazepines in children. It is usually easier to find a psychological explanation for anxiety in children than it is in adults, and the concept of the person biologically predisposed to anxiety has not been explored. It would seem reasonable that occasional doses of benzodiazepines might be useful in children refractory to other measures.

## ATTENTION-DEFICIT/HYPERACTIVITY DISORDER
### Diagnostic Considerations

A child with attention-deficit/hyperactivity disorder (ADHD) may be inatten-tive and restless in class. During recess he may fight with a classmate. He may have difficulty learning to read, spell, or write numbers. His thinking may be poorly organized. His behavior may be impulsive. He may be clumsy and inept at sports. What ails him?

Each of these symptoms, among others, has been identified as part of this vague disorder of children, which has elicited a variety of names. They may also be the symptoms and signs of a normal but neglected child; or a child with mental retardation, schizophrenia, or depression; or a child with specific learning disabilities; or perhaps a child with frequent petit mal epileptic attacks. Obviously, such a confusing assortment of disorders is not easily separated by casual observation. Diagnosing such disordered behavior in children challenges the mettle of the most skilled child psychiatrist.

The teacher may be the first to recognize symptoms and signs of learning disability and poor social behavior. Parents are often loath to see any abnor-mality in their children, a natural reaction. Even when it is recognized, they hope that as the child goes to school he will "grow out of it." So it may become the teacher's unpleasant, but helpful, job to raise the issue of diagnostic referral. And generally the teacher can provide exceedingly valuable observations for evaluating the results of treatment.

Sometimes the diagnosis is easy. The child is driven by an uncontrollable urge to move, purposelessly and continually. He races from one idea to another, without being able to sustain his attention. These two symptoms, increased activity and distractability, are the primary components. The diagnosis may be made a little more secure if the electroencephalogram (EEG) proves to be abnormal, although an abnormal EEG alone is not diagnostic. So-called "soft" neurologic signs may also be present: mild visual or hearing impairments; crossed eyes or fine, jerky lateral eye movements; poor fine visual-motor coordination; confusion of laterality, with frequent left-handedness.

This syndrome of unknown cause is found in about 3 per 100 school children in the United States. Estimates vary between geographic areas and socioeconomic groups, being higher in urban poor than in suburban middle-class children. Boys are affected several times as often as girls, for reasons not clear. The disorder is worldwide, although some countries claim to have an exceedingly low prevalence. A degree of brain dysfunction, based either on genetic or environmental conditions, is assumed, but not proved. For many of these children, psychological or social factors may be more evident than biologic causes.

Although it was formerly believed that children "outgrew" the disorder at puberty, mounting evidence suggests that it persists not only through adolescence but into adult life. About 50 percent of children diagnosed with this disorder show the same symptoms in adult life. Antisocial behavior also seems to be excessive in the grown-up children (Cantwell, 1985; Gittelman et al., 1985). Thus, a diagnosis of attention-deficit disorder, residual type, has been recognized.

## Treatment with Drugs

### Stimulants

For no other childhood psychiatric disorder has drug therapy been more extensively studied nor more definitely shown to be of value. Yet even at this writing, the use of drugs for treatment is highly controversial. During the 1930s, it was observed that some "hyperkinetic" children improved remarkably when treated with amphetamines. This observation has been repeatedly confirmed over the past 50 years. Yet we have little idea of the mechanism by which stimulant drugs mitigate (paradoxically, it has been said) the hyperactivity that is a crucial part of the syndrome.

All psychostimulants are catecholomimetics; they promote the release, block the reuptake, and inhibit the metabolism by MAO of both dopamine and norepinephrine by various degrees. Their chemical structures may be compared to the catecholamines and a prototypical monoamine inhibitor, tranylcypromine, in Figure 7-1.

The pharmacology of dextroamphetamine has been best studied, and in-depth reviews are available elsewhere (Kuczenski, 1983). First, dextroamphetamine is more effective in releasing dopamine than norepinephrine, whereas at higher concentrations it blocks the reuptake of norepinephrine more effectively than dopamine. However, this curious dissociation of its effects on catecholamine release and reuptake may be explained by understanding the molecular mecha-

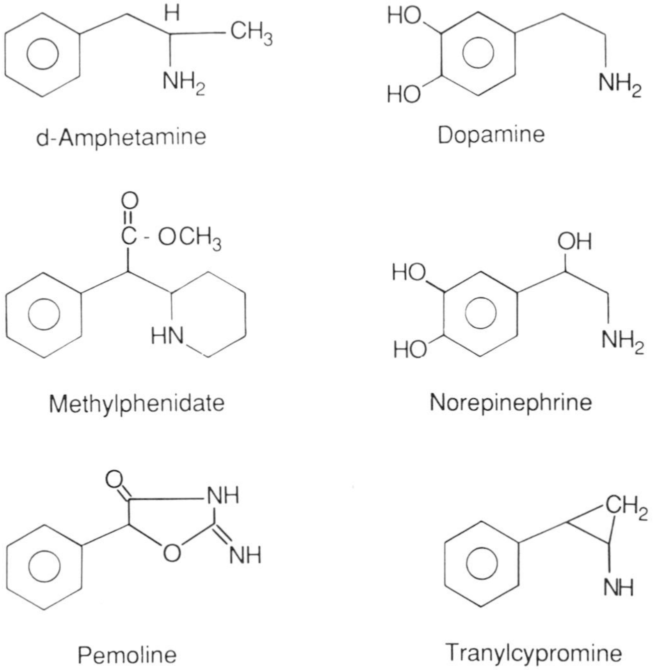

**Fig. 7-1.** Psychostimulants and related compounds.

nism(s) of action of the drug. The catecholamine-releasing actions of dextroamphetamine are independent of calcium, indicating that this process is distinct from the normal depolarization-triggered exocytotic release of neurotransmitter. Rather, it is believed that dextroamphetamine-induced dopamine and norepinephrine release occurs because of a reversal of the reuptake mechanism.

This hypothetical process is illustrated in Figure 7-2. When dextroamphetamine appears in the synaptic cleft, it is transported via a carrier molecule into the presynaptic terminal by the catecholamine reuptake mechanism. However, this causes a disproportionate number of carrier molecules to appear on the internal surface of the cell membrane, and because the concentration of dopamine in the cytosol of the presynaptic terminal far exceeds the concentration of dextroamphetamine, dopamine is transported out of the presynaptic terminal in turn. Only neurotransmitter in the cytosol that has not already been taken up into secretory vesicles is available for such exchange; this may explain dextroamphetamine's greater capacity to release dopamine over norepinephrine. Dopamine beta-hydroxylase, the enzyme that converts dopamine to norepinephrine in norepinephrine neurons, is an intravesicular enzyme (Kuczenski, 1983).

Higher concentrations of dextroamphetamine are required to effectively block the catecholamine reuptake mechanism in both dopamine and norepinephrine terminals. Dextroamphetamine also has acute effects on MAO and may increase

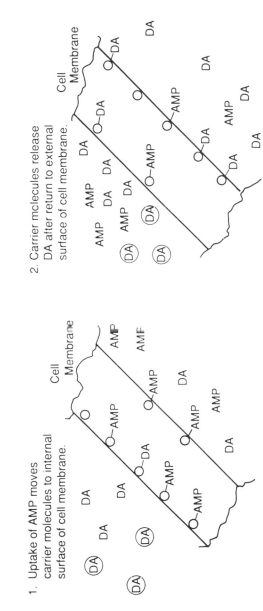

1. Uptake of AMP moves
   carrier molecules to internal
   surface of cell membrane.

2. Carrier molecules release
   DA after return to external
   surface of cell membrane.

**Fig. 7-2.** Mechanism of dopamine release by dextroamphetamine. AMP, d-amphetamine; DA, dopamine.

the cytosolic pool of dopamine and norepinephrine by disrupting vesicular storage.

For most of the past 25 years, the dextroamphetamine surrogate methylphenidate has been the preferred stimulant for this use. The preference is largely based on the fact that methylphenidate has been less widely abused than amphetamines. Yet there are few to recommend between the two drugs in terms of efficacy and safety. A third stimulant, magnesium pemoline, has also been shown to be effective, but for various reasons it has not become popular.

There are some differences in the pharamcologic effects of menthylphenidate and magnesium pemoline compared to dextroamphetamine. However, the pharmacology of these other psychostimulants has not been studied with equal depth. In addition, the pharmacology of cocaine, although it is never used to treat attention-deficit hyperactivity disorder, is obviously related to the pharmacology of dextroamphetamine. In brief, methylphenidate is as potent or more so than dextroamphetamine in inhibiting the reuptake of dopamine and norepinephrine in vitro; in clinical practice it is definitely less potent. Its ability to release catecholamines is weak compared to dextroamphetamine, and the mechanism of this effect is still ambiguous (Kuczenski, 1983). Biochemical studies of magnesium pemoline suggest that its effects are almost entirely dopaminergic.

The efficacy of psychostimulants for decreasing the cardinal symptoms of ADHD is well substantiated. In addition, however, treatment with dextroamphetamine has also been shown to improve classroom behavior (Abikoff and Gittelman, 1985) and increase the acquisition of academic skills (Pelham et al., 1985; Douglas et al., 1986). In many of these studies, children with the syndrome could no longer be distinguished from controls after treatment. The overall efficacy of methylphenidate appears to be equivalent compared to dextroamphetamine, at least in terms of relieving the cardinal symptoms of the syndrome. Its potency is less, so that usual doses are twice those of dextroamphetamine (Gittelman, 1983). The efficacy of magnesium pemoline has also been documented (Conners and Taylor, 1980), although some consider its effects not to be as clear-cut (Gittelman, 1983).

An area of continued controversy is whether the beneficial effects of dextroamphetamine in childhood ADHD occur because of a nonspecific tranquilizing effect peculiar to children. In other words, dextroamphetamine might be expected to have this effect in all children, regardless of whether they had ADHD or not. In one study, all boys, whether or not they carried the diagnosis, reported feeling "tired" or "different," and had lower ratings of motor activity after taking dextroamphetamine. In contrast, normal adult males reported euphoria and had no change in ratings of motor activity (Rapoport et al., 1980). Thus, the results of this study suggest that stimulants would be useless in treating adult attention-deficit hyperactivity. However, both methylphenidate (Mattes et al., 1984; Wender et al., 1985) and magnesium pemoline (Wender et al., 1981) were found in fact to be efficacious in adults with this syndrome.

Sometimes response to drugs can be used as a diagnostic test. If the response is favorable, and this will usually be quickly apparent, then one assumes that the diagnosis is correct. Failure to respond to stimulants occurs in one-third to one-half of ADHD children. This high failure rate may be due to misdiagnosis, inadequate use of the drugs, or to the fact that the syndrome has multiple causes. After all, our behavioral repertoire is finite and the same symptom, restlessness, may be seen in a wide variety of emotional and neurologic disorders. Some children who fail to respond to stimulants may later respond to other drugs, such as tranquilizers and antidepressants, which would imply misdiagnosis.

Daily doses of dextroamphetamine range from 2.5 to 40 mg. After a single oral dose of 0.45 mg/kg, peak plasma concentrations of 63 to 66 ng/ml can be achieved after 3 to 4 hours. The elimination half-life of dextroamphetamine after this single oral dose is 6.8 hours (Brown et al., 1979). Therefore, dextroamphetamine is usually given in divided doses throughout the day. Daily doses of methylphenidate usually range from 5 to 80 mg/day, and again are divided as needed. After a single oral dose of 0.3 mg/kg, peak serum concentrations occur at approximately 1 hour and vary widely among individuals (1.3 to 24.2 ng/ml, mean 12.8); the elimination half-life ranges from 2 to 4 hours (Gualtieri et al., 1982). Pemoline has an appreciably longer half-life, so that it may be administered as a single daily dose (37.5 to 112.5 mg) in the morning.

Many years of clinical use of psychostimulants in children with this disorder should have alleviated fears about safety, but some still persist. Anorexia and insomnia would be anticipated from known pharmacologic actions. Anorexia diminishes with continued treatment, and insomnia may respond to an altered dosage schedule. Weight loss and growth suppression can occur during treatment, but both adverse effects are rapidly reversible when the drugs are stopped. Most children attain their anticipated stature despite treatment (Golinko, 1984). Recurrent fears are that exposure early in life to drugs that might be subsequently abused might lead to increased dependence on stimulants during adult life. Considering the extent of antisocial behavior that seems to be part of the disorder in adult life, it would appear that the prevalence of drug abuse in treated children is less than what might be expected. Occasionally, children treated with stimulants develop tics resembling Tourette syndrome.

## Tricyclics

Imipramine has been used fairly regularly as an alternative drug treatment for ADHD. In controlled studies, imipramine has been reported to be superior to placebo. Yet its efficacy does not equal that of stimulants, and its side effects are more frequent (Rapoport et al., 1974). Sedation is the most common side effect, and sympathomimetic-like side effects, such as decreased appetite and increased blood pressure, may be seen as well. Although imipramine should be tried in children who fail to respond to or cannot tolerate stimulants, it is not a first-line drug. Desipramine, which is a selective uptake inhibitor for norepinephrine, has been shown to be effective. Thus, it is possible that this neurotransmitter is involved in the pathogenesis of the disorder (Donnelly et al., 1986).

Some clinicians believe that tricyclics may be more effective for controlling hyperactivity and impulsivity, whereas stimulants do more to alleviate the attentional disorder. Therefore, combination treatment may have merits.

"Drug holidays" were often the custom in the past, with all drugs being stopped during vacation periods when affected children were out of school. The assumption was that parents might be less bothered by the aberrant behavior than the school class. However, many parents have found that continued treatment may improve the quality of life for the family. If discontinuation of stimulants leads to regression in the attentional disorder, this is of less consequence when school is not in session. Past reticence to use tricyclics was due to the fact that having these drugs around young children has led to accidental overdoses. It is possible that newer, safer antidepressants, such as buproprion, may be preferable (Casat et al., 1987).

## Other Approaches to Treatment

Treatment with the MAO inhibitor clorgyline had an immediate beneficial effect comparable to that of dextroamphetamine during a crossover 4-week treatment trial. The immediate effect from the MAO inhibitor was different from the usual delay in response when these drugs are used for treating depression (Zametkin et al., 1985). The apparent efficacy of clonidine lends further support to a noradrenergic mechanism (Hunt et al., 1985). The suggestion made a few years back that dietary constitutents, especially salicylates and food colorings, were the cause of hyperactivity has been investigated by a number of defined diets. Although some reports suggested minimal benefit, the current consensus is that diets have no role to play in treatment (NIH Consensus Conference, 1982).

It has been traditional to view drug therapy as only a portion of the entire treatment program, with primary emphasis on special classes, perceptual-motor training, and, for those children with secondary effects from their disorder, psychotherapy. However, even drugs alone may provide improved classroom behavior and enhanced academic achievement. A linear dose-response to methylphenidate and measures of these criteria of improvement were demonstrated, independent of any other intervention (Pelham et al., 1985). Similarly, a 16-week cognitive training program added nothing when compared with a group who received no training, both groups receiving concurrent stimulants. With placebo substitution, most children required remedication, regardless of previous exposure to cognitive training (Abikoff and Gittelman, 1985). Nonetheless, it seems reasonable not to restrict treatment solely to drugs.

Some of the most ardent advocates of drug treatment of this disorder are the parents of children who have had it. A favorable response to treatment favorably affects the entire family. On the other hand, periodically, the present being one of those times, controversy over the use of stimulant drugs becomes agitated. Obviously, no one should initiate treatment with any drug in children without the full assent of the parents.

# AUTISM

## Diagnostic Considerations

The child seems singularly detached, staring not at you but through you. He never speaks but often cries or grunts unintelligibly. He avoids human contact, preferring to sit in a corner rocking or flapping his hands before his face. If a top is available, he will spin it incessantly. He is extremely resistant to any change of routine. Such are the manifestations of autism.

This disorder of childhood has remained a mystery ever since its first description. It remains one of the most devastating psychiatric diseases of infancy and childhood. A few decades ago, most theories that sought to explain the illness were psychological in nature. The behavior of parents, in most cases the mother, was thought to cause the appearance of the extreme social withdrawal and self-preoccupation seen in autism. This may have been due in part to the fact that when Leo Kanner first described the disorder in 1943, cases of autistic-like behavior combined with evidence of intellectual deficit were not included within the diagnostic category (Kanner, 1971). Autism was only diagnosed when no evidence of "organicity" could be found. Thus, this notion almost preempted clinical evidence that autism could be due to a pathologic process in brain and encouraged comparisons between autism and other "functional" disorders of childhood, such as schizophrenia.

The diagnosis is based almost totally on behavioral symptoms, as no physical abnormalities have been clearly defined. For many years, autism was classed with childhood schizophrenia. More recently, our understanding of autism and its relation to other developmental diseases has changed. A firmer boundary has been established between infantile autism and schizophrenia (see earlier). Moreover, assumptions that infantile autism may not be accompanied by intellectual deficit have been discarded. In fact, the great majority of cases of infantile autism diagnosed today are known to be accompanied by findings of cognitive deficit (DeMyer et al., 1981). In the DSM-IIIR, the term for this illness is now *autistic disorder*. The name itself suggests that this syndrome may be caused by a variety of brain insults; the modifier "infantile" has been dropped. A comprehensive list of behavioral disturbances (see Table 7.2) now defines the diagnosis, and few exclusionary criteria, including age of onset, are stated. Even if the cause is known, such as would be the case with congenital rubella infection, the diagnosis of autistic disorder could still be applied. Today autism is generally considered to be a developmental disorder of the brain.

A popular notion to explain autism is that the left brain is underdeveloped or damaged (which may account for the intellectual deficit) while the right brain may actually overcompensate (which may result in some remarkable restricted abilities along the lines of idiot-savants) (Blackstock, 1978). However, the variety of manifestations and degrees of impairment do not readily fit any single model. Some autistic children, who retain intellectual functions and attain

## Table 7-2. Criteria for the Diagnosis of Autistic Disorders

A.
- — Marked lack of awareness of the existence of feelings of others
- — No or abnormal seeking of comfort at times of distress
- — No or impaired imitation
- — No or abnormal social play
- — Gross impairment in ability to make peer friendships

B.
- — No mode of communication
- — Markedly abnormal nonverbal communication
- — Absence of imaginative activity
- — Marked abnormalities in production of speech
- — Marked abnormalities in form or content of speech
- — Marked impairment in ability to converse, despite adequate speech

C.
- — Stereotyped body movements
- — Persistent preoccupation with parts of objects
- — Marked distress over changes in trivial aspects of environment
- — Unreasonable insistence on following routines in precise detail
- — Markedly restricted range of interests and preoccupation with one narrow interest

D.   Onset during infancy or childhood

At least eight of the above items are present, these to include at least two items from A, one from B, and one from C.

Modified from DSM-IIIR (1987) American Psychiatric Association, Washington, DC

language, may have a relatively favorable prognosis. Those with IQ levels below 70 rarely do well.

## Response to Treatment

Neuroleptics, such as haloperidol, have long been used in the treatment of autistic children. The daily doses tend to be smaller than those that are used to treat psychosis in children or adults. In one classic study, haloperidol was found to be effective in decreasing symptoms of interpersonal withdrawal as well as stereotypic behavior (Campbell et al., 1978). Interestingly, a variety of more "nonspecific" symptoms, such as hyperactivity and anger, did not respond. Although these effects were seen most clearly in older children within the sample, the older children tended to take higher haloperidol doses (0.15 mg/kg day). Thus, data such as these argue against the notion that neuroleptics have only a nonspecific tranquilizing effect in autistic patients. The benefit from haloperidol seems to pertain to some of the central deficits of the syndrome. As a follow-up to this study, haloperidol has also been shown to enhance learning and retention of learned material in autistic children (Anderson et al., 1984). In eight patients with early infantile autism and aggressive and self-abusive behavior, beta-blockers (mainly propranolol) were added to existing treatment with antipsychotics. Doses ranged from 100 to 420 mg/day of propranolol. A decrease in the target behaviors was noted, suggesting that beta-blockers might be "neuroleptic-sparing" (Ratey et al., 1987).

A number of investigators have found elevated levels of platelet serotonin in the blood of autistic children. This finding has led to novel pharmacologic approaches to the treatment of autism with serotonergic antagonists. However, so-called hyperserotonemia is not specific to children with autistic disorder; it is also found with mental retardation and schizophrenia. Thus, it remains unclear whether hyperserotonemia is related in any way to the specific pathogenesis of autism, or whether it is related to the illness in some nonspecific way (Young et al., 1982; DeMyer et al., 1981).

Nonetheless, trials of the serotonin-depleting agent fenfluramine have yielded some promising results in autistic children. In a large multicenter study, treatment for several months with fenfluramine (1.50 mg/kg/day) produced robust decreases in blood sertotonin concentrations (no significant change in the platelet count was seen), as well as an improvement in autistic symptoms. Moreover, lower blood serotonin concentrations at baseline predicted a superior drug response (Ritvo et al., 1986). Not all studies of this approach to treatment have been so encouraging. A placebo-controlled study that employed fenfluramine in doses of 1.5 to 2.0 mg/day found no differences between the treatments on the Clinical Global Impression Scale or the Parent-Teacher Questionnaire. Only one item of 19 on another scale, withdrawal, showed some improvement with fenfluramine, but this finding could have occurred by chance (Campbell, 1988). Even those who have reported favorably on the drug note many adverse effects. During the initial 2 weeks of treatment, listlessness, food refusal, and stomach upset were noted; during the final 14 weeks of treatment, irritability, agitation, and crying were noted along with continued food refusal. Patients lost 2.1 percent of initial body weight, although a rebound weight gain followed cessation of treatment (Realmutto et al., 1986).

With the uncertain benefits of drug therapy, much reliance is still placed on various psychotherapies. Behavioral techniques are most widely employed. Attempts are made, by use of various rewards, to shape desired behaviors and eliminate those that are undesired. Various more direct educational approaches have also been used. The progress of autistic patients is often measured in extremely small increments. For whatever reasons, a rare patient seems to obtain enough benefit from the various approaches to treatment so that one is encouraged to continue to try to ameliorate the situation even in the face of initial discouragement.

# MENTAL RETARDATION

While each passing year brings new insight into some cause of mental retardation, the majority of cases still are of unknown cause. Furthermore, the range of disabilities is tremendous, so that some patients with modest degrees may function relatively undetected in normal society whereas others must be institutionalized for life. In the absence of any secure knowledge of the cause of most cases, all treatment, whether it be drug or psychosocial, is directed mainly at the alleviation of symptoms.

In general, the milder the degree of retardation, the more emphasis is given to various rehabilitative techniques, aimed at allowing the patients to function better in society. These include education about various daily activities of living, supervision of elementary homemaking skills, and vocational training aimed at placement in some undemanding but necessary job. Such patients seldom require drug therapy unless they also happen to suffer from a concomitant psychiatric disorder.

On the other hand, more severe forms of mental retardation are often accompanied by a marked behavioral change, including constant agitation, yelling, disrobing, incontinence of urine and feces, or self-mutilation. Although behavioral techniques may be useful for some symptoms, much greater reliance must be placed on treatment with drugs. Thus, the majority of institutionalized mentally retarded are treated with one or another psychotherapeutic drugs, often being on multiple drugs. Patients who are most likely to receive drugs in institutions are those in smaller institutions, women, and those with a diagnosis of psychosis (Tu and Smith, 1979). Probably the greatest factor determining the use of drugs is the philosophic bent of the staff. Thus, psychosocially minded staff are much more likely than not to see patients as over-medicated.

Most experience with medication has revolved around use of antipsychotic drugs. They have been used alone, or in combination with sedatives, principally for behavioral control. On the other hand, it is possible that sedation may further impair the ability of patients to learn new techniques of adaptation. The dangers of tardive dyskinesia following prolonged use of antipsychotic drugs have also reinforced conservatism not only in selecting patients for treatment but also in the doses of drug used.

Experience with lithium is less, but it may have a role to play, if nothing more than as an adjunct to antipsychotics (Sovner and Hurley, 1981). One runs the risk of increasing neurologic complications from such a combination. Whether carbamazepine can be used as an alternative to lithium, as in so many other uses, remains to be seen. High doses of beta-blockers have been used to control agitated, aggressive behavior in adults, but experience in children is lacking. Tricyclic antidepressants have been used in mentally retarded patients with apparent depression or those with phobias (Rothman et al., 1979).

# MISCELLANEOUS DISORDERS
## Conduct Disorder

The diagnosis of conduct disorder is made frequently, in about 4 percent of boys, but its boundaries are not clear. Its hallmark seems to be highly aggressive and explosive behavior. A double-blind comparison of haloperidol, lithium, and placebo was carried out in 61 treatment-resistant (at least to psychosocial interventions) children aged 5 to 13 years. Optimal doses of haloperidol ranged between 1 and 6 mg/day while lithium ranged between 500 and 2000 mg/day. Both drugs were significantly superior to placebo in decreasing behavioral symptoms. Lithium produced fewer untoward effects. The effect of both drugs on cognition was mild (Campbell et al., 1984).

## Enuresis

The efficacy of tricyclic antidepressants, especially imipramine, for treating enuresis has been well established since the 1960s. Both effects on the bladder due to anticholinergic and sympathomimetic actions of the drug as well as changes in the architecture of sleep have been adduced as mechanisms for the efficacy of such treatment. Usually, single doses of 25 to 50 mg given at bedtime suffice. Unfortunately, benefits are obtained only as long as the drug is given and are rapidly lost when it is discontinued. Tolerance to the beneficial effects may develop in some patients (Rapoport et al., 1980). For these reasons, many pediatricians like to try alternative, behaviorally based techniques of treatment before resorting to tricyclics (Stewart, 1975).

## Anorexia/Bulimia

The relationship between anorexia and bulimia, and of both with depression, has only been recognized during the past decade. Antidepressants, both tricyclics and MAO inhibitors, have been used with some success. A blind comparison of phenelzine and placebo in bulimics clearly demonstrated the superiority of phenelzine (Walsh et al., 1984). Although the patients in this study were all adults, one assumes that similar results might be obtained in the late adolescents who frequently have these problems. Doses ranged between 60 and 90 mg/day of phenelzine.

## Tourette Syndrome

This tic syndrome tends to become manifest early in life, usually during adolescence. Minor variants are increasingly recognized. It is now believed to have a strong genetic predisposition, as it often occurs in families. The exact mechanism is unknown. Fortunately, the dopamine $D_2$ antagonist pimozide has proven to be highly effective. The advantages of pimozide are that it has few of the unwanted pharmacologic actions of other antipsychotics, such as haloperidol, which is also effective. Symptoms usually wane spontaneously as the patient approaches the fourth decade of life.

## Narcolepsy

This paroxysmal disorder is now considered to be much more frequent than formerly believed. Besides uncontrollable sleep episodes, patients may also suffer cataleptic attacks. Stimulants, usually dextroamphetamine, are useful for the sleep attacks, and tricyclics, such as imipramine, reduce the cataleptic attacks.

# REFERENCES

Aakrog T, Mortensen KV (1985) Schizophrenia in early adolescence. Acta Psychiatr Scand 72:422–429

Abikoff H, Gittelman R (1985) Hyperactive children treated with stimulants. Is cognitive training a useful adjunct? Arch Gen Psychiatry 42:953–961.

Anderson LT, Campbell M, Grega DM, et al (1984) Haloperidol in the treatment of infantile autism: effects on learning and behavioral symptoms. Am J Psychiatry 141:1195–1202

Angold A (1988) Childhood and adolescent depression. I. Epidemiological and aetiological aspects. Br J Psychiatry 152:601–617

Annell A (1969) Lithium in the treatment of children and adolescents. Acta Psychiatr Scand 207 (suppl):19–30

Anthony J, Scott P (1960) Manic-depressive psychosis in childhood. J Child Psychol Psychiatry 1:52–72

Arboleda C, Holzman PS (1985) Thought disorder in children at risk for psychosis. Arch Gen Psychiatry 42:1004–1013

Blackstock EG (1978) Cerebral asymmetry and the development of infantile autism. J Autism Child Schizophr 8:339–353

Brown GL, Hunt RD, Ebert MH, et al (1979) Plasma levels of d-amphetamine in hyperactive children. Psychopharmacology 62:133–140

Brumback RA, Weinberg WA (1977) Mania in childhood. II. Therapeutic trial of lithium carbonate and further description of manic-depressive illness in children. Am J Dis Child 131:122–126

Campbell M (1988) Fenfluramine treatment of autism. J Child Psychol Psychiatry 29:1–10

Campbell M, Anderson LT, Meier M, et al (1978) A comparison of haloperidol and behavior therapy and their interaction in autistic children. Am Acad Child Psychiatry 17:640–655

Campbell M, Grega DM, Green WH, Bennett WG (1983) Neuroleptic-induced dyskinesias in children. Clin Neuropharmacology 6:207–222

Campbell M, Small AM, Green WH, et al (1984) Behavioral efficacy of haloperidol and lithium carbonate. A comparison in hospitalized aggressive children with conduct disorder. Arch Gen Psychiatry 41:650–656

Cantwell DP (1985) Hyperactive children have grown up. What have we learned about what happens to them? Arch General Psychiatry 42:1026–1028

Carlson GA, Cantwell DP (1980) Unmasking masked depression in children and adolescents. Am J Psychiatry 137:445–449

Casat CD, Pleasants DZ, Van Wyk Fleet J (1987) A double-blind trial of buproprion in children with attention deficit disorder. Psychopharmacol Bull 23:120–122

Conners CK, Taylor E (1980) Pemoline, methylphenidate, and placebo in children with minimal brain dysfunction. Arch Gen Psychiatry 37:922–930

Cytryn L, McKnew DH (1972) Proposed classification of childhood depression. Am J Psychiatry 129:149–155

Cytryn L, McKnew DH, Bunney WE Jr (1980) Diagnosis of depression in children: a reassessment. Am J Psychiatry 137:22–25

DeMeyer MK, Hingtgen JN, Jackson RK (1981) Infantile autism reviewed: a decade of research. Schizophrenia Bull 7:388–451

Donnelly M, Zametkin AJ, Rapoport JL, et al (1986) Treatment of childhood hyperactivity with desipramine: plasma drug concentrations, cardiovascular effects, plasma and urinary catecholamine levels and clinical response. Clin Pharmacol Ther 39:72–81

Douglas VI, Barr RG, O'Neill ME, Britton BG (1986) Short term effects of methylphenidate on the cognitive, learning and academic performance of children with attention deficit disorder in the laboratory and the classroom. J Child Psychol Psychiatry 27:191–211

Eisenberg L (1964) Role of drugs in treating disturbed children. Children 11:167–172

Feinstein SC, Wolpert EA (1973) Juvenile manic-depressive illness. J Am Acad Child Psychiatry 12:123–136

Fish B, Shapiro T, Campbell M (1966) Long-term prognosis and the response of schizophrenic children to drug therapy: a controlled study of trifluoperzine. Am J Psychiatry 123:32–39

Flament MF, Rapoport JL, Berg CJ, et al (1985) Clomipramine treatment of childhood obsessive-compulsive disorder. Arch Gen Psychiatry 42:977–983

Frommer EA (1967) Treatment of childhood depression with antidepressant drugs. Br Med J 1:729–732

Geller B, Cooper TB, Chestnut E, et al (1984) Nortriptyline pharmacokinetic parameters in depressed children and adolescents: preliminary data. J Clin Psychopharmacol 4:265–269

Gittelman R (1983) Experimental and clinical studies of stimulant use in hyperactive children with other behavioral disorders. pp 205–226. In Creese I (ed): Stimulants: Neurochemical, Behavioral, and Clinical Prespectives. Raven Press, New York

Gittelman R (1985) The normalizing effects of methylphenidate on the classroom behavior of ADDH children. J Normal Child Psychology 13:33–44

Gittelman R, Mannuzza S, Shenker R, Bonagura N (1985) Hyperactive boys almost grown up. I. Psychiatric status. Arch Gen Psychiatry 42:937–947

Gittelman-Klein R, Klein DF (1973) School phobia: diagnostic considerations in the light of imipramine effects. J Nerv Ment Dis 166:199–215

Golinko BE (1984) Side effects of dextroamphetamine and methylphenidate in hyperactive children—a brief review. Prog Neuropsycholpharmacol Biol Psychiatry 8:1–8

Gram LF, Rafaelsen OJ (1972) Lithium treatment of psychotic children and adolescents. Acta Psychiatr Scand 48:253–260

Green WH, Campbell M, Hardesty AS, et al (1984) A comparison of schizophrenic and autistic children. J Am Acad Child Psychiatry 23:399–409

Gualtieri CT, Wargin W, Kanoy R, et al (1982) Clinical studies of methylphenidate serum levels in children and adults. J Am Acad Child Psychiatry 21:19–26

Hunt RD, Minderra RB, Cohen DJ (1985) Clonidine benefits children with attention deficit disorder and hyperactivity: report of a double-blind placebo-crossover therapeutic trial. J Acad Child Psychiatry 5:617–629

Insel TR, Murphy DL, Cohen RM, et al (1983) Obsessive-compulsive disorder. Arch Gen Psychiatry 40:605–612

Kanner L (1971) Followup study of eleven autistic children originally reported in 1943. J Autism Child Schizophr 1:20–32

Kashani JH, McGee O, Clarkson SE, et al (1983) Depression in a sample of 9-year-old children. Arch Gen Psychiatry 40:1217–1223

Kashani JH, Shekim WO, Reid JC (1984) Amitriptyline in children with major depressive disorder: a double-blind crossover pilot study. J Am Acad Child Psychiatry 23:348–351

Kramer AD, Feiguine RJ (1981) Clinical effects of amitriptyline in adolescent depression. J Am Acad Child Psychiatry 20:636–644

Kuczenski R (1983) Biochemical actions of amphetamine and other stimulants. pp 31–61. In Creese I (ed): Stimulants: Neurochemical, Behavioral, and Clinical Perspectives. Raven Press, New York

LaGrone DM (1981) Manic-depressive illness in early childhood. South Med J 74:479–481

Mattes JA, Boswell L, Oliver H (1984) Methylphenidate effects on symptoms of attention deficit disorder in adults. Arch Gen Psychiatry 41:1059–1063

NIH Consensus Conference (1982) Defined diets and childhood hyperactivity. JAMA 248:290–292

Parnas J, Schulsinger F, Schulsinger H, et al (1982) Behavioral precursors of schizophrenia spectrum. ARch Gen Psychiatry 39:658–664

Pelham WE, Bender ME, Caddell J, et al (1985) Methylphenidate and children with attention deficity disorder. Arch Gen Psychiatry 42:948–952

Preskorn SH, Weller EB, Weller RA (1982) Depression in children: relationship between plasma imipramine levels and response. Psychopharmacology 43:450–453

Puig-Antich J, Blau S, Marx MD, et al (1978) Prepubertal major depressive disorder. J Am Acad Child Psychiatry 17:695–707

Puig-Antich J, Perel JM, Lupatkin W, et al (1979) Plasma levels of imipramine (IMI) and desmethylimipramine (DMI) and clinical response in prepubertal major depressive disorder. AM Acad Child Psychiatry 18:616–627

Rapoport JL, Quinn PO, Bradbard G, et al (1974) Imipramine and methylphenidate treatments of hyperactive boys. Arch Gen Psychiatry 30:789–793

Rapoport JL, Buchsbaum MS, Weingartner H, et al (1980) Dextroamphetamine. Arch Gen Psychiatry 37:933–943

Rapoport JL, Mikkelsen EJ, Zavadil A, et al (1980) Childhood enuresis II. Psychopathology, tricyclic concentration in plasma, and antienuretic effect. Arch Gen Psychiatry 37:1146–1152

Rapoport J, Elkins R, langer DH, et al (1981) Childhood obsessive-compulsive disorder. Am J Psychiatry 138:1545–1554

Ratey JJ, Mikkelsen E. Sorgi P, et al (1987) Autism: the treatment of aggressive behaviors. J Clin Psychopharmacol 7:35–41

Realmutto GM, Jensen J, Klykylo W, et al (1986) Untoward effects of fenfluramine in autistic children. J Clin Psychopharmacol 6:350–355

Ritvo ER, Freeman BJ, Yuwiler A, et al (1986) Fenfluramine therapy for autism: promise and precaution. Psychopharmacology Bull 22:133–140

Rothman CB, Chusid E, Giannini MJ (1979) Mental retardation. Behavior problems and psychotropic drugs. NY State J Med 79:709–715

Stewart M (1975) Treatment of bedwetting. JAMA 232:281–283

Sovner R, Hurley A (1981) The management of chronic behavior disorders in mentally retarded adults with lithium. J Nerv Ment Dis 169:191–195

Tu Jun-bi, Smith JT (1979) Factors associated with psychotropic medication in mental retardation facilities. Compr Psychiatry 20:289–295

Walsh BT, Stewart JW, Roose SP, et al (1984) Treatment of bulimia with phenelzine. A double-blind, placebo-controlled study. Arch Gen Psychiatry 41:1105–1109

Weinberg WA, Brumback RA (1976) Mania in childhood. Case studies and literature review. Am J Dis Child 130:380–385

Wender PH, Reimherr FW, Wood DR (1981) Attention deficit disorder ('minimal brain dysfunction') in adults. Arch Gen Psychiatry 38:449–456

Wender PH, Reimherr FW, Wood D, Ward M (1985) A controlled study of methylphenidate in the treatment of attention deficit disorder, residual type, in adults. Am J Psychiatry 142:547–552

Werry JS (1967) The use of psychoactive drugs in children. Illinois Med J 131:785–787

Werry JS (1979) Principles of use of psychotropic drugs in children. Drugs 18:392–397

Whitehead PL, Clark LD (1970) Effect of lithium carbonate, placebo and thoridazine on hyperactive children. Am J Psychiatry 127:124–125

Young YG, Kavanaugh ME, Anderson GM, et al (1982) Clinical neurochemistry of autism and associated disorders. J Autism Develop Disord 12:147–165

Youngerman J, Canino I (1978) Lithium carbonate use in children and adolescents. Arch Gen Psychiatry 35:216–224

Zametkin A, Rapoport JL, Murphy DL, et al (1985) Treatment of hyperactive children with monoamine oxidase inhibitors. Arch Gen Psychiatry 42:962–966

# Index

*Note:* Page numbers followed by f designate figures and those followed by t designate tables.

* Available in generic form.